MEDI
their ori

Ffrangcon Roberts'
MEDICAL TERMS:
their origin and construction

SIXTH EDITION
extensively revised and enlarged by

Bernard Lennox

MD, PhD, FRCP(G), FRCPath.

Emeritus Professor, Department of Pathology
(Western Infirmary), University of Glasgow

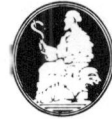

WILLIAM HEINEMANN MEDICAL BOOKS LTD.
LONDON

William Heinemann Medical Books Ltd
23 Bedford Square
London WC1B 3HH

First edition 1954
Second edition 1956
Third edition 1959
Fourth edition 1966
Fifth edition 1971
Sixth edition 1980

This edition copyright © Bernard Lennox 1980

ISBN 0 433 19151 1

Printed and bound in Great Britain by
Morrison & Gibb Ltd., London and Edinburgh

Ff.R. dedicated his book to his daughter Joy,
B.L. dedicates the 6th edition to his wife Mary.

Socrates: Have the courage to admit that one name may be correctly and another incorrectly given; and do not insist that the name shall be exactly the same with the thing. . . . I should be astonished to find that names are really consistent.

PLATO, Cratylus.

Words strain,
Crack and sometimes break, under the burden,
Decay with imprecision, will not stay in place,
Will not stay still.

ELIOT, Burnt Norton.

PREFACE TO THE SIXTH EDITION

Dr Ffrangcon Roberts died in 1977. He was born in 1888 in Bethesda, a doctor's son, went to Epsom College, Clare and Thomas's and married a daughter of Clem Attlee. He was a consultant radiotherapist in Cambridge and of high repute in that capacity: he was also a man of wide learning, noted for his command of English as well as the classics. He seems to have been a difficult man to cross at times, but was in spite of this widely liked and respected. The first edition of this book appeared in 1954, and was recognized at once as filling a unique and useful niche, by helping doctors and those who work with them to a more genuine understanding of the words they used. It remained popular enough to call for four further editions from his pen.

I have no pretensions at all to match Dr Roberts' classical scholarship, my own interests lying rather with the current meanings of medical words and the ways in which they have changed with time. I have accordingly interfered very little with the word lists which are the centre-piece of the book: idiosyncratic though the choice and arrangement may seem, they have delighted and educated many thousands of readers, and their content is timeless. Elsewhere I have reorganized it very extensively, including many of my own ideas, but the best of the original is preserved in the new text. Only part five is wholly mine. My own views on such things as Latin and Greek plurals and the authority of etymology in deciding the meaning of a word are a good deal more radical than his, but I hope that he would have recognized I am only reflecting a continued shift in opinion on these matters, which in turn reflects the continuing increase of importance of English as an international means of communication.

I have to thank the editor of the *Lancet* for permission to base parts of section 5 on material contributed to that journal. I must also acknowledge that nearly all the information on the etymology and older history of words that I have added to this book is derived from the Oxford English Dictionary, and that without the willingness of its current editor, Robert Burchfield, to listen to my views on the current meaning of medical terms, I would never have had the impertinence to try and teach my contemporaries anything about the words they use.

I must thank too the many colleagues who have discussed the use of medical terms with me over the years, and especially Dr A. T. Sandison, who read the manuscript for me, and also Mrs Pat Bonnar, most long-suffering of secretaries.

B. L.

FROM THE PREFACE TO THE FIRST EDITION

The great majority of those studying medicine, whether as medical students, nurses or auxiliaries, come to the subject with no knowledge of the classics. They are therefore compelled to learn, or rather to pick up, a vocabulary which is entirely new to them and which is extremely complex. Under the circumstances it is remarkable how well they succeed. Nevertheless I believe that their task would be made much easier and their work more interesting if they understood the origin and mode of construction of the words which they read, hear, speak and write.

This book is not a dictionary in the ordinary sense of the term. For the student who wants to find by a short cut the meaning of an isolated medical term many excellent dictionaries exist. In any case the meaning is usually obvious from the context or from direct experience. Here the meaning is given only when it is not clear from the context. I believe that the principles and examples given should enable the reader to deduce the derivation of most words which he is likely to meet.

Ff. R.

CONTENTS

Part I	Our classical roots	1
	English and medical English	
	Dissecting medical words	
	Relics of ancient medicine	
	Examples of classical derivations	
	Greek words in Latin	
Part II	Word-construction	25
	Prefixes and suffixes	
	Examples of word-construction	
	New words	
	On being classically correct	
Part III	Exemplary word lists	45
Part IV	Non-classical origins	89
	Modern French	
	Italian	
	Spanish	
	German	
	Arabic	
	Others	
	Acronyms	
	Eponyms	
Part V	Miscellany	103

ABBREVIATIONS

Ant., antonym.
Adj., adjective.
Ar., Arabic.
E., modern English.
F., modern French.
Fem., feminine.
G., Greek.
Gen., genitive.
L., Latin.
Lit., literally.

M.E., Middle English.
O.E., Old English.
O.E.D., Oxford English Dictionary.
O.F., Old French.
Orig., originally.
Pl., plural.
Pop., popular.
Prob., probably.
Syn., synonym.

Foreign words are Greek unless stated otherwise.

TRANSLITERATION

The representation of Greek letters in English presents some difficulty and, at best, can only be conventional. There is no way of distinguishing the Greek short σ (omicron) from the long ω (omega); the Greek rough breathing can only be rendered by the letter h; γ before the gutturals γ, κ, χ, ξ, which was pronounced n, must be rendered by n. I have aimed at simplicity rather than orthographic accuracy, despite the inconsistency which results. I have rendered the Greek κ usually by c, but sometimes by k, whichever is the nearer to English usage; similarly the Greek v sometimes by y and sometimes by u. χ is rendered by ch, and ξ by x.

PART I

OUR CLASSICAL ROOTS

The purpose of medical language is to describe, as simply and unambiguously as possible, the facts of medicine we can recognize and the ideas which we have formed concerning them. The language must be adaptable and expandable in order to keep pace with the constant multiplication of these facts due to new methods of examination and treatment, and with the perpetual revision and evolution of our concepts. It gives us a verbal picture of the ideas concerning disease which civilized man has entertained over the last 2,500 years. It illustrates the changes in the concepts of disease which the years have brought, and incidentally it gives us interesting glimpses of the lives which our progenitors lived.

We must admit at the outset that, as compared to the symbols used in mathematics and the physical sciences, the verbal symbols used in medicine, as in most of biology, are often imprecise. This imprecision arises in part from the fact that, in the sciences dealing with living matter in general and living people in particular, one is so often describing behaviour of great complexity which is imperfectly understood. Often also we are using words originally devised for some new idea which fit it imperfectly when time and newer knowledge have changed the idea out of recognition. In many older words one can detect a substratum of ancient and irrational systems of medicine, and in many recent ones an element of the surviving belief in the magical power of a name to give one control over something one does not understand. None of this absolves anyone from the duty to use words as exactly as possible.

THE LIMITATIONS OF THE VERNACULAR

At all times and in all countries people have found ways to describe their medical experiences and their views about them which have been confined within the limits of everyday speech. So long as the subject-matter is simple this may be adequate and even poetic: "He fell off from the seat backwards by the side of the gate, and his neck broke and he died; for he was an old man and heavy." (I Sam. iv, 18)

By reason of its simplicity and directness this passage might well serve as a model for a medical witness at an inquest – at least as a preliminary statement that the jury could follow. As soon as the witness was asked for precise information as to what had happened to Eli's neck, he would be in trouble. "A breaking-off of the tooth-like knob of the second bone from the top of the spine of the neck, the one upon which the head turns" is a clumsy way of describing a fracture of the odontoid. 'Ordinary' words reflect the standard of knowledge of the 'ordinary' man, and their use to express the more exact knowledge of the expert in any field involves long-winded paraphrases. This does not concern medicine only: see how much longer that last sentence becomes if you try to replace "paraphrases" with simple everyday words and get the whole of its sense across.

The good honest old words, mostly of Anglo-Saxon origin, that form the back-bone of English have two other disadvantages. One is their limited capacity for joining together to form the compound words needed to express complex ideas. (Of course this may be partly from lack of practice: if we had no alternative we might see nothing wrong with words like liverbignessdisease or withinwindpipe-unfeelingness: German accepts such words almost too readily.) The other is the fact that such words, though often readily understood by other northern Europeans, have no such wide international currency as have words derived from Latin and Greek. In practice, the vast majority of the specialized words of medicine are derived in some way from the classical languages, and this applies nearly as much to words of recent coinage as to the old words, in spite of the fact that those who coin them may often have little or no knowledge of the original tongues.

It happens that these two languages (and especially Greek) are well adapted for the purpose, but the reason for their use in this way is a matter of historical accident rather than design. It was obviously a very complicated process, but it is worth trying to trace the gist of it.

ENGLISH AND MEDICAL ENGLISH

THE MIDDLE AGES. After 1066 there were three languages in England – the Norman-French of the ruling group, who usually held land in France as well as England; the Latin of the churchmen, lawyers and a few other scholars; and the mix of Anglo-Saxon dialects with some Danish and other oddments spoken by the oppressed majority. During the next two centuries, without written literature to stabilize it, the Old English of this oppressed majority sensibly altered, becoming simpler and more flexible. When King John lost Normandy, the aristocracy lost their French connexions and began to count themselves English, and came to use English more and more. When Richard II addressed Wat Tyler's rebels in English, it was something notable: Henry V, a generation later, was more at home in English than French (though perhaps not to the extent that Shakespeare so comically pretended). These new recruits greatly expanded and embellished the language they adopted.

By 1400 the emergence of a powerful, sophisticated and often courtly literature, of which Chaucer's *Canterbury Tales* is the best-known representative, served notice that a new language was coming into full flower. The same thing was happening to northern dialects (witness the marvellous *Sir Gawain and the Green Knight*) and to Lowland Scots (witness Henryson and Dunbar), but it was the language of

East Anglia and London, of the Court and Chaucer and Wyclif's Bible, and (though they taught in Latin) of Oxford and Cambridge, that was most affected and formed the basis of modern English.

French vanished, but many of its words remained. English had been the language of the low and the illiterate, and when the rulers and the learned shifted from French to English, they found it necessary to take with them many French words, words especially of administration and the law, of fighting and hunting, of good living and luxuries, and of abstractions and literature – combining these with the older elements to build up a massive new vocabulary.

The doctors of the time made the same change, and carried medical words already current in French with them into English – medicine, physician, surgeon, pleurisy, gout, poison and many others. Most such words came to French from Latin. It is usually impossible just by looking at a word like 'medicine' to say whether it came into English directly from Latin or via French: only after discovering when such a word first occurs in English, how it was used and how it was spelled at that time, can one know the truth about its history.

We have thus a massive infusion of words, Latin in origin but often Old French in form, into English before 1400, and some of these were medical, the earliest and smallest of the three main contributions of the classical language to medical English.

THE LATIN OF SCHOLARS. Through all this time Latin remained the international language of the Church, of scholars generally, and of diplomacy; scholars could wander from Aberdeen to Vienna, from Bologna to Stockholm, listening to lectures, reading manuscripts, defending propositions, all in Latin. Ambassadors parleyed and treaties were written in it. No learned doctor, whether of medicine or theology, would dream of writing in any other tongue. And this continued for a long time: Harvey wrote *De Motu Cordis* in 1628, and the translation

On the Circulation of the Blood did not appear till 1653. It was not until after 1700 or thereabouts that Latin ceased to be usual for medical works. (The chief aim of an Oxbridge medical education in the 1700s was said to be the ability to read Galen and Hippocrates in the original, nor should we laugh too loudly at this, for it is not so long ago that Latin ceased to be compulsory for entrants to medical schools in this country.)

The factors that conspired to break this monopoly of Latin as the scholar's language during the century or so beginning about 1540 were many. The rise of prosperous nation states with pride in their own language and their own new literature was perhaps the chief. The Reformation rejected the Latin of the Roman church and encouraged instead bibles and copious theological works in the vernacular. Luther's Bible (1521) was the making of modern German, and Coverdale's (1535) almost as important for English. Printing helped, for printers soon discovered there was more money in long runs of popular works for the multitude than in Latin treatises for scholars. The discovery that fellow citizens like Dante, Shakespeare and Cervantes could write as well as the ancients, that Columbus, Da Gama and Drake could enlarge the world, that Vesalius, Copernicus, Galileo and Harvey could make brilliant and fruitful discoveries of things unknown to all the old philosophers, broke the belief that all true art and all true wisdom could be found in the classics.

The Renaissance, against all expectations and intentions, had the same effect. Better knowledge of the originals showed that a great part of the learning in the Latin texts could be better studied in the original Greek (and sometimes Hebrew), which at one stroke halved the standing of Latin and doubled the amount of work needed to become a true classical scholar. More insidious was the Renaissance scholars' determination to improve the standard of Latin. Mediaeval Latin was a relatively flexible language, readily adaptable to the many new purposes that had been found for it. The new men insisted that the grammar must be that of Cicero: no word not found in the classical authors was admissible. The result was the dead language of School Certificate Latin, useless for normal communication.

Note this as an awful warning: the dead hand of legislators, grammarians, dogmatic dictionary-writers, Academicians and old gentlemen who write letters to *The Times* makes for a dead language. Only use, which is always changing, defines a language.

Latin died, but, like Norman-French, its words lived. Scholars and the new breed of scientists, switching from Latin to English, had to take the words of their trade with them. Poets and other literary men, rejoicing in the new freedom of their language, joined in the game. Men like Shakespeare and Ben Jonson and Bacon adopted and adapted words with great freedom, either directly from Latin, or indirectly via Italian and French. English became quite suddenly modern English. For all the expansion and superficial adaptation of the last 300 years, major change has proved unnecessary since the days of Milton and Pepys.

Doctors were slower to adapt themselves than most others. They have always tended to believe that medical knowledge should not be made too readily available to the general public, and writing in Latin was one way of ensuring this. Andrew Boorde published his *Breviarie of Health* in 1547, but he had few followers in the next century. Yet there was a rapid diffusion of medical words into English during this time, far more than those coming earlier via Norman-French. Words like *retention* and *fracture* were introduced into English from Latin as medical terms (in 1400 and 1612 respectively) and taken into general use afterwards.

THE WORD COINERS. This process of adoption into English of words taken from Latin and Greek continued for a long time, and has not altogether ceased yet. The most useful Latin words were soon nearly exhausted, and Greek became a more popular source, only a little devalued by the fact that many Latin words, in the sciences especially, were Greek in origin (see p. 24). But there was a new difficulty: ideas were appearing that classical authors knew nothing about, and had no words for. New words were needed.

Sometimes a Latin word could be adapted in a new sense that was an acceptable extension of the old. 'Circulation' meant originally much the same as rotation (i.e. travel in a circle round a fixed central axis). Harvey extended the word to cover travel round a complex closed circuit – expressing so the core of his great discovery – and this new sense was at once adopted in English by his followers. The old sense has been all but lost, and instead we have another example of a word used originally (in this sense) in a purely medical technical sense and then given wide general currency. Not only blood circulates now, but cash and traffic and ideas. Something the same must have happened with Newton's take-over of the word *gravity* for a wholly new idea.

With increasing confidence people began to make up new words using Latin and Greek rather as models of how to construct words than as direct sources. This process is now overwhelmingly the main source of new words in science. In medicine it has become a flood, baffling those unfortunate lexicographers who have to try to keep up with it, yet, in so far as the new words reflect new ideas (and mostly they do) they are a welcome index of advancement of learning in our subject.

MODERN WORD-MAKING. Earlier coiners of words copied their models slavishly, making up words in either Latin and Greek according to the rules followed by the ancients (the Greeks were particularly good at word-making) and then converting to English. Though in fact as far as is known there was no such word for 'within a vessel' as '*intravascularis*' in Latin, it is one that Cicero or Virgil might well hve accepted: hence 'intravascular'. That was fine as long as all educated men could be assumed to know Latin and (if possible) Greek. Nowadays, however, we make up our words directly, often with no reference to classical grammar.

What has happened is that the parts of Latin and Greek have become living elements of the English language. Intravascular, as we have seen, is a copy of what would have been a good Latin word. But our language has adopted 'intra' and 'vascular' as English word elements, to be built up with other adopted elements in accordance with the rules of *English* word formation. We can cheerfully mix Greek and Latin now in formations like intrahepatic and hypervascular, and tolerate such triple mixtures as under-vascularized (Anglo-Saxon prefix, Latin stem, Greek suffix -ize, Anglo-Saxon past tense ending). It is a free, easy and infinitely useful process.

There are, of course, other ways of forming new words, apart from building them out of Latin and Greek elements: some of them are considered in Part IV. But even today, the old classical roots are by far the commonest constituents of new medical terms.

DISSECTING MEDICAL WORDS

Just as a blackbird is not simply a black bird, or a yellowhammer a yellow hammer, one cannot tell always with confidence the exact meaning of a medical term (especially the older ones) from its elements. *Orthopaedics*, which literally means 'straightening of children' (p. 109) is a good and relatively recent example. But in most cases a knowledge of the elements gives valuable clues to meaning, and is a great help to the memory.

Let us take one fairly complex example of a newish word that is familiar enough from many articles about coronary artery disease – *hypercholesterolaemia*. There are six recognizable elements in this, one Arabic and the rest Greek, but most people would divide it into three – 'hyper-' (too much), 'cholesterol' (name of a substance) and '-aemia' (blood) – i.e. 'raised blood cholesterol'. This is an example of what is now a heavily used convention: the name of a substance, followed by '-aemia', and preceded by 'hyper-'

or 'hypo-' (too little) is a universal method of indicating the state of excess or deficiency of that substance in the blood. Since the substances that can be measured in the blood are already numerous, and appear to be added to daily, the number of existing or predictable words so formed is very large. So standard and accepted is this convention that if you discovered tomorrow a disease caused by excess of krypton in the blood, you not only could but would be expected to christen it hyperkryptonaemia at once without ceremony. (Note that in doing so you would be risking confusion between the mere excess of krypton in the blood, and a disease of which that was a characteristic: it is a risk, however, that is generally disregarded.)

'Hyper-cholesterol-aemia' is an easy dissection. But two of the elements can be taken apart further. The familiar *haem* element of so many blood words has lost its h (on the analogy of *anaemia*, which is the original Greek form), and the *-ia* is a vague Greek ending indicating that it is not literally blood itself but some condition connected with it that is in question. Cholesterol is more complex. *Chole* is bile, *ster* is solid (as in stereoscopic – cholesterol is the solid in bile that causes most gallstones) and *ol* indicates that it is chemically an alcohol (an Arabic word greatly changed in meaning from its original Arabic sense). Except for the relation to bile this knowledge is not much help: but it is worth noting that the whole important group of the steroids (cortisone, aldosterone, many sex hormones) owe their name to their chemical resemblance ('oid') to (chole)sterol, which was the first one to be recognized.

It will be seen that the process of understanding a word from the parts of it is by no means easy. But in a large number of cases simple dissection of the hyper-cholesterol-aemia type is readily made and immediately useful if you know the elements.

Before going on to consider the present-day state of the art of constructing words, let us look more closely at the words we have taken over more or less unaltered from classical sources.

RELICS OF ANCIENT MEDICINE

Words have a great capacity for survival. They persist throughout the centuries, long after the things and ideas they stood for and even the languages in which they were first used have become obsolete. Many of them are visible records of outworn concepts. It will be useful at this point to consider some aspects of the ancients' ideas on disease which are still relevant to the words we use today.

GRAECO-ROMAN BELIEFS. Let us try to put ourselves in the place of a doctor living 2,500 years ago. We must divest ourselves completely of all knowledge of chemistry, physics, biology and pathology, and look at the phenomena of disease with the eyes of people with no scientific knowledge. We must imagine ourselves without the stethoscope and thermometer, not to mention more elaborate instruments, unable to look inside the thorax and abdomen during life, and with few opportunities for post-mortem examination. It was a time of great thinkers, but also a time when observation was unimportant and trial by experiment was not to be thought of. A few, like Hippocrates and Aristotle, made genuine observations, but even Aristotle could confidently assert that women had fewer teeth than men, and that to cure an elephant of insomnia the ears should be rubbed with olive oil, salt and warm water.

In these circumstances how should we have explained a cold in the head, coughing of blood, an abdominal tumour or a case of insanity? We should have been forced either to attribute them to the malevolence of the gods, or to construct theories entirely unsupported by evidence. Moreover, mental disturbance playing, as it still plays, a prominent part in practice, we should have had to explain it in terms of the current philosophies concerning the relation between mind and matter.

SOMA, PSYCHE AND PNEUMA. To the Greeks there were three fundamentals of human life; *soma, psyche* and *pneuma*. *Soma* was the body in its material aspects, a meaning which it retained, e.g. *somatic, chromosome* (coloured body). The distinction between *psyche* and *pneuma* was at first confused. Though, in the Iliad, *psyche* means breath, it was mythologically regarded as the personification of the human soul, foreshadowing its present application to the mental component of life in *psychology, psychiatry*. Like psyche, *pneuma* meant soul or spirit and also breath, afterwards the active principle which animated and controlled the whole body. This conception was considerably elaborated by Galen, who described three kinds of pneuma. The blood, reaching the liver from the intestines, was there endowed with the first pneuma: Natural Spirit. This was carried to the right ventricle and thence distributed by the veins to the whole body which it provided with nourishment. Part of the blood reaching the heart passed from the right to the left ventricle through pores in the interventricular septum which were too small to be visible. In the left ventricle it became mixed with blood arriving from the lungs charged with a second pneuma, Vital Spirit, which was distributed to the tissues endowing them with power. Part of this blood passed to the brain where it became endowed with the third pneuma, the pneuma of the soul, or Animal Spirit. This passed along the nerves, which he believed to be hollow tubes, and gave the body the power of movement and feeling. The idea that the blood moved to and fro in the vessels persisted until Harvey discovered the circulation of the blood in 1628. The term pneuma has now been narrowed down to relate only to respiration, e.g. *apnoea* (absence of breathing), *hyperpnoea* (excessive breathing), *pneumonia* (cf. F. *poumon*, lung).

THE HUMORAL THEORY. From Greek times until relatively recently medicine was dominated by what now seems to us an incredible tissue of nonsense, the humoral theory. It was believed that there were four body-fluids: *haima*, blood; *phlegma*, phlegm or mucus; *chole*, yellow bile and *melaina chole,* black bile (biliverdin-stained infected bile, perhaps, or multiple pigment stones). The relative amounts of these determined the temperament, and disease was attributed to gross disturbance in their balance. Excess of blood caused the sanguine (*sanguis,* blood) temperament; excess of phlegm caused the cold, unexcitable, phlegmatic; excess of yellow bile caused the choleric or irascible; excess of black bile caused the melancholic or atra-bilious (*ater,* black). Since black bile was supposed to be formed in the spleen, this organ was associated in common speech with spite and ill-humour, e.g. 'to vent one's spleen'. The use of humour for a fluid is retained in the aqueous and vitreous humours of the eye.

The humours could also become overheated, *Zeein,* boil, appears in *eczema,* lit. boiling out, and, in combination with *kara,* head, in *coryza,* which to us means "cold in the head". The nasal secretion was supposed to come from the base of the brain through the skull and was called *pituita* (mucus or phlegm). Hence, ultimately and most curiously, the *pituitary*.

Rheumatism is an especially odd humour product. *Rheum* originally was an alternative name for the phlegmatic humour. It once was used in English for a cold, and 'rheumy' eyes (chronically watering) are still occasionally heard of. But a theory that joint disease was due to excessive 'flowing of the humours' produced *rheumatism*: hence came the names of two genuine (and quite different) diseases, *rheumatic fever* and *rheumatoid arthritis*. Rheumatism is left with no real sense at all except a vague association with painful joints.

FEELINGS AND EMOTIONS. The idea that feelings and emotions arise in organs other than the brain persists in many ways. From the frequent reference of imaginary pains to the upper part of the abdomen we get *hypochondria* – 'below the rib cartilages'. *Phrenic* (phrenic nerve, *phrene,* mind) conveys the same idea. *Hysteria* (*hystera,* womb) perpetuates the belief that in women the origin of functional disorders may be associated with uterine abnormalities. Let those who may be amused at these notions reflect upon their own habit of attributing the emotions to the heart.

Of the function of nerves the Greeks were ignorant. They used *neuron* both for nerves and tendons, and, as Galen taught, they believed the nerves to be hollow. Though *neuron* now means a nerve cell and forms the basic word in *neurology*, the older and wider connotation persists in *aponeurosis*, tendinous sheet.

Sympathetic (nerves) is difficult. According to the O.E.D., the first reference (and that an indirect one) is dated 1769, where it is described as synonymous with 'intercostal'. The originator and the reason are unknown. It has nothing to do with the ordinary harmony-of-feeling sense common to modern English and ancient Greek.

EXAMPLES OF CLASSICAL DERIVATION

Innumerable names are derived from resemblance to Roman buildings, animals and plants or their parts, or to their musical instruments, articles of adornment, agricultural implements, tools and wepons. Here we shall confine ourselves to the general principles involved.

An open space for assembly or marketing was called *agora* (hence *agoraphobia*, fear of open spaces). An enclosed space, if large, was called *claustrum* (*claustrophobia*, fear of being shut in), and, if small, *areola* (*areolar* tissue, i.e. tissue of small spaces). In a house, the vestibulum led into the *atrium* (to us synonymous with *auricle*). This may have been so-called because it had a fire in the middle of the room and therefore had blackened walls (*ater*, black). An inner room or bedroom in Greece was called *phragma* (hence diaphragm) in Greece and *septum* in Rome. The fireplace was called *focus*, hence the modern meaning – centre of heat and light. A beam (in the roof) was called *trabs*, dim. *trabeculum*. Passages were called *fauces*. A gate-keeper was called *pylorus* (the pylorus guards the entrance to the small intestine).

Outside there would be *via*, road, *fornix*, arch, *stylos*, pillar (styloid process). Water was conveyed by a *ductus*, *fossa* (ditch), *fistula* (pipe) or *cloaca* (sewer). There would also be the *latrina*. A large house would have a fountain, *fontana*, in the court, hence *fontanelle* (dim. through F.), possibly from the pulsation on an infant's head's resembling bubbling. If the owner possessed a vineyard he would have a *torcula* (wine press). Among the domestic utensils were *penicillia* (brushes) and *cribra* (sieves). *Porta*, entrance, appears in portal vein, so-called by Galen because he considered the transverse fissure to be the entrance to the liver.

Examples of musical instruments are *salpinx*, trumpet, *tympanum*, drum; of articles of adornment, *fibula*, brooch, *peroneus*, tongue of a brooch; of agricultural implements, *vomer*, ploughshare, *falx*, scythe; of tools, *malleus*, hammer, *incus*, anvil; *stapes*, stirrup; of weapons, *ensis*, sword (*ensiform*, sword-like). A body of soldiers in close order was a *phalanx*: the fingerbones in their regular rows form a phalanx, but the name is now applied to them individually.

In many of the above examples, the resemblance is fairly remote or fanciful, and sometimes an addition is made to the word to signal this.

1. With (usually) Greek words, *-oid* (G. *eidos*), as in *colloid*, glue-like.
2. With (usually) Latin words, *-iform*, as in *vermiform*, worm-like.
3. With (usually) Greek words, *para-*, as in *paratyphoid*. (A resemblance at two removes: typh*oid* was once thought to be only a variety of typhus, and *para*-typhoid is a close relative of typhoid.)
4. By the prefix *pseudo-* (*pseudes*, false).

ASSOCIATION

Frequently the device is employed of naming a thing from a thing or idea associated with it. This takes several forms:

1. The material or animal used.
    Histology, from *histos*, woven material.
    Vaccination, from *vacca*, L. cow.
    Graft, from *graphein*, write, through O.F. *graffe*, F. *greffe*, M.E. *grift*. The Gauls were taught the art of horticultural grafting by the Romans, the slips used being shaped like pencils.
    Inoculation. Originally this also meant a gardener's grafting, the bud to be grafted being the 'eye' (*oculus*). Cf. the eye of a potato.

2. An attribute.
    Anopheles, harmful (insect).
    Sacrum, L. This bone was considered sacred and was used in sacrificial rites. Since it was the last bone to decay it was believed that the body would re-form around it.
    Jejunum, L. empty, because it is empty after death.
    Cornea, L. horny. Originally *tela cornea*, horny tissue.
    Caecum, L. Blind.
    Decidua, fem. adj., falling off; *membrana* is understood.
    Melaena (*melaina*), fem. of *melas*, black (originally accompanied by the fem. noun *nosos*, disease).
    Lumen, L. light; hence something which transmits light, i.e. a clear space.
    Duodenum, L. twelve inches (in length).

3. The use of an organ.
    Thenar. *Theinein*, to strike; striking being one of the uses of this part of the body.
    Buccinator. L. *bucina*, trumpet. Muscle of cheek used in blowing a trumpet.
    Sartorius. *Sartor*, tailor. Muscle used in crossing the legs.

4. A characteristic of a substance or animal.

Anthrax and **carbuncle** (L. *carbo*) both mean coal, the characteristic being burning. John of Trevisa (1535), translating the great mediaeval encyclopaedia, *De Proprietatibus Rerum,* by Bartholomeus Anglicus, a book probably used by Shakespeare, has: "Antrax is a postume whyche cometh of ful wood matere and venomous. It is callyd also 'carbunculus' for it brennyth like a cole."

Alopecia. from *alopex,* fox, the characteristic being manginess. Trevisa, from the same source, has: "By that euyll callyd Allopicina nourysshynge of heer is corrupte and fayllyth, and the foreparty of the heed is bare, such men fare as foxes."

5. Indirect association.

Quinsy from *cyon,* dog, *anchein,* throttle, through O.F. *squinancie* and F. *esquinancie.* The idea was no doubt derived from the self-strangulation of a dog straining at the leash. At first it was applied to any obstruction of the throat.

Idio-, in *idiopathic, idiosyncrasy* means peculiar to oneself. In Greek times *idiotes* meant a private person, private in the sense that he kept himself to himself and took no part in public affairs. Such behaviour was considered contemptible. Hence it came to mean inexpert or ignorant and this is the origin of *idiot.*

Carotid, *caros,* sleep, because compressing these arteries produces unconsciousness (cf. F. *garrotter*).

Pupil (of the eye), L. *pupilla,* little girl or doll, from the small image of oneself seen in another's eye. *Glene,* the Greek word for pupil, means mirror and conveys the same idea, but it also means a shallow cavity and appears in this sense in *glenoid.*

Myopia, *myein,* to close, *ops,* eye, from the way short-sighted people screw up their eyes.

Pudenda, L., external genitals, from L. *pudere,* to be ashamed.

Thorax, orig. breast-plate. Transferred to the part covered by a breast-plate.

Climacteric, *climakter,* rung of a ladder. The critical year. The seventh and its multiples were considered critical years, the grand climacteric for men being the sixty-third year, 7 by 9.

Oestrus, gadfly, a modern word. In some animals sexual excitement resembles the excitement due to a sting.

SPECIFIC USE OF GENERAL TERMS

It has always been customary, before the true nature of a disease is known, to describe it from its most prominent symptom. *Fever* has been used through the ages for many different conditions. P.U.O. (*pyrexia of unknown origin*) is the modern form which this confession of ignorance takes. As diseases become differentiated, a term which was originally applied to a group becomes permanently attached to a single member of the group.

Morbilli, L. measles, from L. *morbus,* disease; also *rubeola,* red.

Typhus (*typhos,* smoke or mist) was a figurative way of expressing the stupor of mistiness of vision caused by fever in general.

Eclampsia (*ek,* from *lampas,* light) was used by Hippocrates for any illness arising suddenly like a flash of light. The idea may, however, have arisen from the flashes of light supposed to be seen by the patient.

Glaucoma (*glaucos,* greyish-green) was applied to any condition in which the eye was of a greyish colour.

Halitosis is derived from L. *halitus* which means breath or vapour in general; it now means a state of bad breath.

Herpes (G. creep) was applied to any spreading condition.

Hypopyon which originally meant any local infection, is now limited to suppuration of the anterior chamber of the eye.

Leprosy. Lepra originally meant any scaly condition of the skin.

Hymen originally meant any partition.

'Attacks.' Our incorrigible habit of blaming anything or anybody but ourselves for our misfortunes leads us to accuse the environment of raining attacks, blows and strokes upon our offending persons. We have 'an attack' of indigestion when out own indiscretion is almost certainly the cause. So it has always been. Medical literature abounds in the idea: *impetigo*, from L. *impetere*, attack; *epilepsy, catalepsy*, from *lepsis*, attack; *plague, monoplegia, paraplegia, hemiplegia*, from *plege*, blow.

GENERAL USE OF SPECIFIC TERMS

Examples of this are fewer:

Epithelium possibly meant the surface over the nipple (*epi*, upon, *thele*, nipple) or other projecting areas. Together with the cognate word *endothelium* and the more recent *mesothelium* it is now applied to surfaces of all kinds.

Nausea (*naus*, ship) in early Greek times meant sea-sickness, but by the time of Hippocrates it had acquired its modern sense.

MAJOR SHIFT OF SENSE

Sometimes words have undergone such marked changes of senses as to be barely recognizable: they can be reversed or even carry two opposed senses at once.

Asphyxia, absence or weakness of the pulse (*a*, neg., *sphyxis*, pulse), acquired its modern meaning in the eighteenth century.

Atheroma (*athere*, porridge) meant sebaceous cyst, from the character of the contents. Its transfer in the nineteenth century to aortic disease was no doubt due to the somewhat similar appearance.

Arachnoid, resembling a spider or spider's web. Hippocrates used *arachnoides* for scum on urine; Galen, for a venous or nervous plexus. The modern meaning dates from the seventeenth century.

Cele (swelling) was applied to a swelling of any kind whether due to a tumour, hernia or other cause. The term was later restricted to swellings containing fluid: *cystocele, hydrocele, haematocele, meningocele* (not *coele* – see p. 116).

Condyle (*kondylos*, knob) at first meant both knuckle and exostosis before being applied to certain projections of bone. *Condyloma*, a venereal wart.

Parenchyma (*para*, beside, *en*, in, *chyme*, juice; pouring in of juice). A term invented by Erasistratus (300 BC) to express his view that the blood was carried into the organs and there congealed. The word now means the cells specific to an organ as distinguished from the fibrous stroma and blood vessels.

Nystagmus, orig. drowsiness, hence the nodding of the head in drowsiness: now only abnormal rhythmic eye movement.

Cataract meant not only a waterfall or rapids but the obstruction to the river which produces the rapids, or even a sluice-gate. Hence the sense of something which *obstructs* vision. Ambroise Paré (1550) calls it in French a '*cataracte ou coulisse*' (*coulisse* = portcullis).

Hippus, orig. winking, equivalent to nystagmus; now altered to contraction and dilatation of the iris.

Tarsus, orig. flat basket, extended to any flat surface including flat of the foot and tarsal ligament of the eye: then transferred from flat of the foot to the bones.

Phlegmatic means cold or indifferent, though derived from *phlegein*, burn. The contradiction, however, is more apparent than real. The Greeks regarded nasal catarrh as a typical example of inflammation or burning. The result of this burning was discharge of phlegm which Hippocrates in *The Nature of Man* describes as the coldest of the humours.

Symposium, which now means a learned discussion, in Greek times meant drinking-party. High thinking was, however, far from being neglected. If we can trust Plato's

Symposium (one of whose participants was a doctor), the Greeks got more inspiration from their wine-cups than we get from our tea-cups.

Valgus originally meant bow-legged; it now means the opposite.

Nyctalopia (*nyx, nycto-,* night, *alaos,* blind, *opsis,* sight) has from ancient times been used and is still used in two opposite senses; night-blindness and, by disregard of -al-, night vision or better vision at night. Galen uses it in the former sense but quotes Hippocrates as using it in the latter. Similarly *hemeralopia* (*hemera,* day) is used in both senses: day-blindness and better vision by day. These words should be confined to their etymological meaning: *nyctalopia,* night-blindness and *hemeralopia,* day-blindness.

OBSCURE ORIGINS

Abdomen, L. origin unknown, but possibly related to adipose, fat.

Abscess, L. *abscessus,* gone away (i.e. the contents).

Acne, prob. corruption of *acme,* point.

Amnion meant lamb and also bowl for receiving the blood of sacrificial animals. Its first application to a fetal membrane appears in the writings of Empedocles of Agrigentum (504–443 BC), but there is no reason to suppose that he connected this use with either of its other meanings, capable though he was of supersonic flights of imagination.

Aorta (*aorter,* strap), used by Hippocrates for the bronchi.

Astragalus had no less than eight meanings. Both in the *Iliad* and in the *Odyssey* it is used for one of the upper cervical vertebrae. It also meant a knuckle-bone. Hippocrates uses it for what is now known as the talus. It seems to have been applied to any bone used for gambling. Dice were, in fact, called *tali*. For this purpose the Greeks favoured the first or second cervical vertebrae while the Romans favoured the talus.

Cretin may have been derived from F. *cretin*, a corruption of *chretien*, Christian. If so, the reason is not clear. It may have been a term of contempt for Christians. The word, however, also meant a human creature as distinguished from a beast. The term would thus imply that cretins were human despite their animal appearance. Another explanation is that Christians were driven by persecution to the remote valleys where they developed cretinism. This seems unlikely, since these valleys contained pagans as well.

Fomes, L. pl. *fomites*, now used for clothing, etc., capable of carrying infection. In L. it means touchwood.

Hernia, L. prob. from G. *hernos*, sprout.

Hydatid, probably watery vesicle.

Keloid, variously attributed to *kele*, swelling, *kelis*, blemish, and *chele*, claw of a crab or hoof of a horse.

Lupus, L. wolf (reason unknown).

Mydriatic (*mydros*, cautery). The connexion is obscure. The idea may have been that dilatation of the pupil could be caused by fear of the cautery.

Os Innominatum. L. No name could be found for it.

Peristalsis (*peri*, around, *stellein*, to place), used by Hippocrates for contraction.

Rickets. Much disputed. It was certainly a new word for a newly discovered disease in the mid 1600s. Evelyn the diarist says it was named after an 'empiric' (i.e. quack) of Somerset called Rickets who first described it. There is no other record of his existence. A medical description of 1645 calls it *rhachitis* (from *rachis*, spine) – on the face of it an odd name, as the spine is not the most obviously involved bone structure. A middle English word, *wrikken*, to twist, has also been suggested, again with little evidence.

Temple, temporal. Prob. related to L. *tempus*, time. G. *temnien*, cut?, cut off in time?, a good place for striking; or perhaps because the greying of the hair shows the passage of time.

Thymus (*thymos*, thyme) was at first applied to any warty excrescence, from the supposed resemblance to a bunch of thyme. It was first used for the gland by Galen. The name suggests sweetness, and English butchers sometimes call it neck-sweetbread to distinguish it from the pancreas, but the idea that sweetness is the connexion is far-fetched. *Thymos* with a different pronunciation (and certainly a different word) meant soul or feelings. Hence the modern word *cyclothymia*.

Vitiligo. *Vitis.* L., vine, or *vitium,* blemish.

MYTHOLOGICAL

Some of the names derived from mythological figures are of great antiquity, but many have been added recently by psychologists who have discovered in ancient literature prototypes of abnormal behaviour.

Adam's Apple. According to tradition this marks the place where the fruit given to Adam by Eve stuck in his throat.

Aphrodisiac, a drug stimulating sexual desire; from Aphrodite, the Greek equivalent of Venus.

Atlas, so-called because it holds up the head. Atlas was a Titan compelled by Zeus to hold the heavens on his shoulders. The bone was so named by Vesalius.

Atropine (*a, tropos,* no turning – inflexible). Atropos was the Fate who cut the thread of life.

Caesarean section. Julius Caesar was supposed to have been born in this way.

Caput medusae. The dilated veins radiating from the umbilicus in portal obstruction. Medusa was one of the Gorgons. Her hair was turned into serpents by Athene.

Erotic, sexual, from Eros (pronounced *air-rose* not *ee-ross*), another Greek god of love, corresponding to the Cupid of the Romans.

Hermaphrodite, an individual of indeterminate sex. Hermaphroditus was the son of Hermes and Aphrodite. He became physically united with the nymph Salmacis.

Hygiene, from *Hygeia* (health), one of the daughters of Aesculapius.

Hymen, Hymen, god of marriage.

Lesbianism Sexual relations between women. Lesbos, an island in the Aegean, the abode of Sappho the poetess, who was addicted to this practice.

Morphia. Morpheus, god of dreams. Note that this is the same word as *morphe,* form, Morpheus determining the form which dreams took.

Narcissism, excessive vanity and introspection. Narcissus, a beautiful youth who thought his image in a fountain was a nymph. On trying to reach it he was drowned.

Oedipus complex, perverted love of one's mother accompanied by hatred of one's father. Oedipus Tyrannus killed his father and married his mother, Jocasta.

Panacea. a cure-all. Panacea was one of the daughters of Aesculapius.

Priapism. Priapus, god of procreation.

Psychology, Psyche, goddess of spirit.

℞ (Recipe). This sign, which precedes prescriptions, is the oldest of all medical signs. It is said to be the contracted form of the eye of Horus. Horus was a god of health in early Egyptian times (about 6000 BC). It has passed through a succession of forms of which ℞ is the latest.

St Anthony's Fire (St Anthony, b.AD 251). This term was, and sometimes still is, applied to erysipelas, but was more probably applied to ergotism, since a burning sensation is a prominent feature of this disease. Ergotism was very common; it was due to infection of rye bread.

St Vitus's Dance. Before his martyrdom in AD 303 St Vitus prayed that all who commemorated his death should be protected from dancing mania. This affliction occurred in epidemic form in Western Europe throughout the middle ages. The term is now confined to chorea.

Syphilis. In 1495 syphilis made its first appearance in Europe having been brought to Naples, it is believed, by the crews of Christopher Columbus's ships. In 1530 Fracastoro, a Veronese physician and poet, wrote an account of it in the form of a poem entitled *Syphilis sive*

Morbus Gallicus (Syphilus or the French disease. The Italians blamed the French for its introduction). In the poem Syphilus is the name given to the patient, a shepherd. The name may have been derived either from *sus,* hog and *philos,* love, i.e. swineherd, or from *syn philos,* accompaniment of love.

Tendo Achillis. To make him invulnerable Achilles was dipped in the river Styx by his mother, Thetis. The heel by which she held him was not submerged. He was killed by a wound in this part.

Venereal, from Venus, Roman goddess of love.

GREEK WORDS IN LATIN

It is sometimes a help to recognize the Greek words which have been altered on adoption into Latin. Very often no change was made, but two kinds of changes were common:

To conform with Latin grammar, endings were often changed:

The ending *-os* in Greek masculine words became *-us, bronchos, bronchus.*

The ending *-e* of Greek feminine nouns became *-a, theke, theca.*

The ending *-on* of Greek neuter nouns became *-um, cranion, cranium.*

The ending *-a* of neuter nouns remained *-a, coma, coma.*

Examples of words so treated are: *aorta, arteria, brachium, bronchus, canthus, carpus, clitoris, colon, gluteus, lochia, limbus, meconium, meninges, oesophagus, perineum, pylorus, radius, retina, tarsus, urachus.*

Many Greek words, in which the initial letter is represented in English by *h,* in Latin begin with *s*:

hemi, semi; hexa, sex; hepta, septem; hyper-, super-; hypo-, sub-.

PART II

WORD-CONSTRUCTION

We must now take up in more detail the reverse of the process exemplified in Part I by our analysis of *hypercholesterolaemia*, and look at the general process of building up words from two or more separate elements. It is a mistake to believe that a knowledge of the classical languages is necessary for this. It is a help if one wants to understand some of the less logical rules of the game, and perhaps also if one finds the existing stock of word-elements already adopted insufficient for one's new ideas. The author of the present edition, however, who retains only a little of his O-level Latin and has never learnt Greek, finds this no great handicap in discussing the *present-day* use and construction of words.

STEMS. All but the simplest words have a central component, the stem, to which other elements are joined. Most medical words have stems of classical origin – of this numerous examples are given in the previous section and in Part III. We are chiefly concerned here with the way prefixes and suffixes are added to these stems. Note, however (and here a little school Latin helps), that the stem often does not correspond to the common dictionary form of the word from which it is taken – not *nox*, (night), but *noct-*, from *noctis:* hence *nocturnal* and *nocturia*. It is best identified as follows:

In both Greek and Latin nouns by the genitive which may be quite different from the nominative:

Nominative	*Genitive*	*Stem*
odous, tooth	*odontos*	*odont-*
pes, L. foot	*pedis*	*ped-*

In Latin verbs by the past participle passive:

Indicative	Past participle passive	Stem
sto, stand	status	stat-

In Greek regular verbs by the future active:

Indicative	Future active	Stem
lyo, to loose	*lyso*	lys-

In Greek irregular verbs it is simpler to take the substantive formed from them:

rhegnynai, to burst	*rhexis, rhagia*, a bursting
temno, I cut	*tome*, a cutting
trepo, I turn	*tropos*, a turning

LINKING VOWELS. When the second component of a word begins with a consonant, linkage between stems is provided:

In Greek words usually by *o*, rarely by *i* or *a*:

Nominative	Stem	Combined form
derma, skin	*dermat-*	dermat-o-logy
neuron, nerve	*neur-*	neur-i-lemma (*lemma*, husk)

In Latin words by *i* or *o*:

dens, tooth	*dent-*	dent-i-gerous
cerebrum	*cerebr-*	cerebr-o-spinal

When the second component begins with a vowel, linkage is unnecessary:

orchis, testis	*orchid-*	orchid-ectomy.

ELISION AND ASSIMILATION. When a word beginning with a vowel or h has a prefix ending in a vowel, this vowel is suppressed:

meta-haemoglobin, methaemoglobin; epi-ulis (oulon, gum) epulis.

Exception: *peri: periarteritis, periosteum.*

An unfortunate effect of this rule is a tendency to mispronunciation by the illiterate. There is no 'th' sound in met-haemoglobin or polycyt-haemia. Insistence on this is not pedantry: the meaning is affected. Meth-aemoglobin would not be a meta- but a methyl derivative of haemoglobin. (A ridiculous converse error occasionally heard is 'parat-hormone'!)

When a prefix ends in a consonant, the consonant is sometimes changed to the consonant with which the following word begins.

    ad-ferent, afferent   *in-ruption, irruption*
    ad-glutinate, agglutinate   *ob-caput, occiput*
    ex-ferent, efferent

    n before a labial *b*, *m* or *p* becomes *m*: *en-bolus, embolus*
    n before *s* is suppressed: *syn-stole, systole*

PREFIXES AND SUFFIXES

LIVE AFFIXES. Very many of the words of medicine are constructed by affixing to the stem one or more standard additions, either before (prefixes) or after (suffixes). Most of those that are used with any frequency are 'live', in the sense that they have been adopted into the English language and may be used freely when needed. A few that have been included in the lists below, such as *ad-* and *epi-*, are doubtfully live – that is to say relatively few readers are aware of the sense they are meant to convey. Those which are names of things and therefore stems in their own right (*gastro-*, *haemo-*, for instance) have not been included except (e.g. *pyo-*, *histo-*) where the sense is not obvious.

The list is intended for rapid reference and gives only minimal definition. The origins of many of them will be found among the lists in Part III of the book (use the index if necessary), in some cases with notes on their usage.

PREFIXES

a, an-	absence	angio-	vessel
acro-	extremity	ante-	before
ad-	towards	anti-	against
adeno-	gland	apo-	away
agno-	unknown	auto-	self
allo-	other	bi-	two
ambo-	both	bio-	life
amphi-	both	brachy-	short

Prefix	Meaning
cata-	down
chole-	bile
cryo-	cold
crypto-	hidden
deutero-	second
dextro-	right-hand
di-	two
dia-	through
dolicho-	long
dorsi-	back (of body)
ecto-	outer
endo-	inside
epi-	upon
erythro-	red
eu-	favourable
ex-	out of
extra-	outside
giga	giant, $\times 10^{12}$
hemi-	half
hetero-	different
histo-	tissue
homeo, homoeo-	similar
homo-	same
hypo-	too much
hypo	too little
juxta-	near
iatro-	medical
idio-	self
infra-	below
inter-	between
ipsi-	self
iso-	same
kata-	down
kilo-	$\times 10^{3}$
laevo-	left-hand
lepto-	thin
macro-	large
mega-	large, $\times 10^{6}$
megalo-	large
meso-	middle
meta-	change
micro-	small, $\times 10^{-6}$
milli-	$\times 10^{-3}$
mono-	single
multi-	many
myo-	muscle
nano-	dwarf, $\times 10^{-9}$
neo-	new
non-	negative
normo-	normal
oligo-	few
ortho-	straight
oxy-	acid, sharp
pachy-	thick
pan-	total
para-	beside
per-	through
peri-	surrounding
pico-	small, $\times 10^{-12}$
pleo-	diverse
pluri-	many
poly-	many
post-	behind, after
pre-	in front, before
proto-	first
pseudo-	false
pyo-	pus
recto-	straight
retro-	behind
rheo-	flowing
sclero-	hard
semi-	half
sesqui-	one-and-a-half
stereo-	three-dimensional, solid
sub-	under
super-	above, too much
supra-	above (position only)
telo-	distant
tera-	monstrous, $\times 10^{9}$
ultra-	beyond
ventri-	front (of body)
xeno-	foreign
zoo-	animal

NUMBERS OVER TWO (GREEK FIRST)

3	tri, ter-	8	oct-
4	tetr-, quadr-	9	ennea-, non-, nov-
5	pent-, quinqu-	10	dec-, decem-
6	hex-, sex-	100	hect-, cent-
7	hept-, sept-	1000	kilo-, milli-

SUFFIXES

Suffixes are liable to modification to form different parts of speech (radio-graph, -graphy, -graphic, -grapher): in general only the shortest form has been given, except where the change of sense is outside the ordinary modifications. The sense is intended to cover the general meaning of all the forms.

-affine	affinity	-ol	alcohol
-agogue	secretion-stimulant	-ology	science
-algia	pain	-oma	tumour
-ase	enzyme	-ose	sugar
-blast	embryonic	-osis	disease
-cele	fluid-containing swelling	-osmia	ability to smell
		-ostomy	forming an opening
-clast	breaking	-otomy	cutting
-cyte	cell	-pathy	disease
-ectasis	dilatation	-penia	lack
-ectomy	cutting out	-pexy	fastening
-ergia	movement	-phasia	ability to speak
-geny, -genesis	origin	-philia	attraction
		-phobia	repulsion
-gram, -graph	writing, picture	-plasty	construction
		-praxia	ability to do
-graphia	ability to write	-privia	lack
-gyria	rotation	-rrhage	bursting out
-ia	disease	-rrhaphy	stitching
-iasis	disease	-rrhexis	bursting out
-ics	branch of medicine	-rrhoea	flow
-iform	resembling	-scope	look
-ine	amino compound	-tome	cutting
-itis	inflammation	-tonic	tension
-lysis	splitting	-trophic	nourishing
-megaly	enlargement	-tropic	seeking
-mycosis	fungal	-topic	site
-oid	resembling		

VARIATIONS IN MEANING. Though there are a good number of suffixes and even more prefixes at our disposal, there are always shades of meaning for which nothing suitable presents itself. The result is the existence of what might be called different interpretations of the original sense.

We often, however, find that established usage compels us to accept senses that have little or no relation to the original meaning. This runs throughout science. In organic chemistry *ortho-*, *meta-* and *para-* are distinguishing terms with no relation to the original meaning. Similarly we have *catalysis*, loosening down, and *analysis*, which literally means loosening up but which might equally mean loosening down. (Note that in ordinary speech 'break up' and 'break down' mean the same thing.) There is no real difference in original meaning between the words *epilepsy*, attack upon, and *catalepsy*. attack down; or between *syndrome*, running together, and *symptom*, falling together.

How arbitrary and remote from their classical meaning modern terms may be is shown by the names given to the three body-types or somatotypes. Rotund persons with a tendency to fat are called endomorphs (*endo-*, inner; *morphe*, form); stocky, heavily-muscled persons are called mesomorphs (*meso-*, middle) and tall, thin persons are called ectomorphs (*ecto-*, outer).

A more bizarre example is *anaphylaxis*; the literal meaning (*ana*, up or back, *phylaxis*, protection) does not make sense. Richet and Poitier at first thought of *aphylaxis* (no protection), but as they did not like the sound of this word they decided upon *anaphylaxis*. Etymology gave way to euphony (Acta Allergologica: 5, 178, 1952).

The Greeks themselves gave prefixes the most diverse meanings, *Cata (kata)* for instance, meant *down, against, on, over, through, wrongly, opposite, after, according to, conforming, very like, about*. We have followed this practice, as the following examples show:

dia	through	*diameter*, measure through
	across	*diaphragm*, partition across
	apart	*diastole*, position of heart-walls apart

meta	next to, or beyond	*metacarpals*, beyond the carpals
	change	*metamorphosis*, change in form
	after	*metanephros*, the last kidney to develop
para	beside (in position)	*parathyroid*
	modified	*paratyphoid*, modified typhoid
	disturbance of	*paraesthesia*, disturbance of feeling

EXAMPLES OF WORD-CONSTRUCTION

GENERAL TERMS

Medicine *(medicina)*, science *(scientia*, knowledge) and doctor *(doctor*, teacher) are basic Latin words. *Physic, physician, physicist, physical* and *physiology* are from the Greek *physis*, nature. The wide use of this word exemplifies the fact that the study of disease is part of the study of nature. (A *physicien* in French is a physicist.) *Physis* also means growth (p. 82).

Surgery is shortened from O.E. *chururgery*, derived from *cheirourgia* (*cheir*, hand, *ergon*, work). The O.E. form is retained in the designation of surgical degrees at some universities: M.Ch., B.Chir.

Iatros, the Greek word for physician, is used only in combined forms: *iatrogenic*, of disease caused by medical treatment, and *-iatrics* (see below).

Apothecary, from *apotheke*, storehouse. Apothecaries were first storekeepers, then grocers, then pharmacists (as in *Romeo and Juliet)*, and then (witness Mr Perry in *Emma*) the lowest-ranked general practitioner.

Therapy. *therepeutics*, from *therapeuein*, to heal, to take care of: *physiotherapy*, treatment by 'natural' agencies, e.g. sunlight, heat; *chemotherapy*, treatment by chemicals.

Pharmacy, *pharmaceutical*, from *pharmacon*, drug.

Dose, *dosis*, L. a giving.

Clinic, clinical from *klinikos*, relating to a bed. (Cf. recline.)

Diagnosis from *gnosis*, knowledge, judgement, *dia*, through, about.

Prognosis, knowledge forwards, i.e. predicting. From the same stem we have *gnomon*, judge, which appears in *pathognomonic*, characteristic of a disease.

Aetiology, study of cause (*aetia*, cause).

Branches of medicine are named:
1. By addition of *-logy (logos*, discourse): *gynaecology, gyne*, woman.
2. By addition of *-ics (the G. adjectival form)* or *-iatrics* (see above, *Iatros*): *orthopaedics* (see p. 109 for the children) and *paediatrics* (G. *pais, paidos*, child).
3. By special names: *Hygiene*, from *hygeia*, health (p. 22).

NAMING DISEASES

'Disease', dis-ease, is a very general term for any departure from health of a degree enough to need attention. Disease comes in all sorts of varieties, and each variety is 'a disease'. There are said to be over 20,000, and new ones are still being discovered: it is not surprising that it is hard to find good names for all of them. They vary greatly in the exactitude with which they can be defined: there is little disagreement about what one means by smallpox or cancer of the bronchus, but much more argument than certainty about such diverse things as neurasthenia, traveller's diarrhoea or cleaved (which should be cloven or cleft anyhow) cell lymphosarcoma.

Confusion arises between actual diseases and manifestations of disease. 'Jaundice' for instance is simply a yellow colour of the skin due to bile-staining, and is an *effect* of numerous diseases, not a disease itself. 'Peritonitis' – inflammation of the peritoneum – though dangerous in itself, is again an effect of numerous diseases, or, better, a 'complication'—i.e. an effect of disease which is serious in itself but does not always happen. 'Hypertension' – high blood pressure – may be an effect of disease but equally can be produced by anger or excitement or an injection of adrenalin, with no question of disease at all. Only when qualified by an appropriate adjective (e.g. 'essential', which here means no more or less than 'of unknown cause') can it be counted as the name of a disease – *essential* hypertension.

Disease names fall mostly into four categories:

(a) SIMPLE DESCRIPTIVE WORDS. Most old names (many of them perfectly good names still fully acceptable) are of this type: they usually refer to some conspicuous feature or some fanciful association. *Rabies, plague* and *cancer* are examples of classical origin, *smallpox, scurvy* and *measles* are native products.

(b) COMPOUND WORDS, made by adding specific suffixes to previously existing words – *appendicitis, silicosis, hepatoma*.

(c) NOUN AND ADJECTIVE NAMES. Most modern names are of this kind: exact definition may require two, three, or even four words. *Diabetes mellitus* and *pachymeningitis haemorrhagica* are examples of names surviving in Latin form, but (except among dermatologists) most names are nowadays anglicized – *pneumococcal pneumonia, rheumatoid arthritis, sub-acute bacterial endocarditis,* or unmistakably English – *farmer's lung, weaver's bottom, whooping cough*.

(d) EPONYMS – i.e. names of people, as in Addison's disease and Pott's fracture. These are considered further below (p. 100).

Do not expect too much logic in this. The biologists can usually agree as to what constitutes a species of plant or animal: they have in the 'mule rule' – which states that crosses between species are generally infertile – a guide that though far from universal at least provides a preliminary standard. In diseases definition can only be operational: if it proves *useful* to group cases together under one name, that name is the name of the disease. An old name, be its derivation ever so doubtful or even nonsensical, if everyone knows it, and it stands clearly for a well-defined entity, may well be preferred to more logical alternatives. *Gout*, though gout may not be due to the drops *(guttae)* of poison once supposed to seep into the affected joint, is still preferred to the more logical and internationally better known '*podagra*' (foot-catcher) or the more scientific '*idiopathic hyperuricaemia*' (too much uric acid in the blood, of unknown cause).

The words essential (not related to anything outside), primary (not secondary to anything else), idiopathic (caused by itself) and agnogenic (arising in the unknown) are simply labels attached to the names of diseases of unknown cause. So long as the diseases are genuine entities, and the labels are accepted as confessions of ignorance and not a method of hiding it, they serve a useful function.

DISEASE SUFFIXES

Except for some of the first group, these have all been included in the suffix list on p. 29, but the definitions need expansion.

(a) Many old word-endings survive in disease names, without any recognizable sense. Such are *-ia* (anaemia), *-ism* (rheumatism), *-ismus* (strabismus), *-ago* (lumbago).

(b) **-itis** is now universally accepted as the mark of inflammation. It was originally simply a Greek adjectival ending: *nosos arthritis* meant disease of the joints, *nosos nephritis* disease of the kidneys and so on: the *nosos* was then dropped. Until last century it was still often used for non-inflammatory conditions: indeed, until the nature of inflammation was established securely, such ascriptions must have been doubtful. Now only a few non-inflammatory uses survive, *(osteo)arthritis* the only common one. Where one finds other terminations used for inflammation, one can be sure the word is old – *pneumonia* and *pleurisy* for instance (though pleurisy is a late Latin corruption of Greek *pleuritis*) and new forms of lung inflammation are often called pneumonitis. Note incidentally that -*itis* words may or may not be disease names: most often they are pure descriptive terms, e.g. *meningitis*, needing further definition to become diseases (e.g. *tuberculous meningitis*).

(c) **-osis,** originally a Greek suffix making nouns from verbs, like the -ing in 'drawing' when it means a picture, is now a general-purpose ending meaning a non-inflammatory condition. It is commonest in names indicating the presence of some abnormal collections of material – *silicosis, haemosiderosis, lipidosis*. In *nephrosis* it serves as a direct contrast with *nephritic* and indicates specifically absence of inflammation. So also with *diverticulosis* and *diverticulitis*. It is used also for infections – *tuberculosis, actinomycosis* – even though, as in these two cases, inflammation of a kind may be present.

(d) **-asis** (usually -*iasis*) is merely a variant of -*osis*. It is used now especially for non-bacterial infections, chiefly tropical – *filariasis, schistosomiasis, trypanosomiasis*, where in every case the first part of the word is the name of the infecting organism. (An ancient Greek with lice had *phthiriasis*.) But there are many other uses – *psoriasis*, for example, which originally meant itchiness. Note that these words are all now pronounced with a strong stress on the penultimate i as in filari:-asis.

(e) **-pathy.** (G. *pathos*, suffering, disease). Another neutral disease ending, popular at present amongst pathologists, but with other earlier uses (see p. 106).

(f) **-oma.** On the model of carcinoma, this is used very widely for tumours. Nowadays it is confined to true tumours, but earlier it might be attached to any chronic swelling – hence tuberculoma, granuloma, leproma, trachoma and the like.

NEW WORDS

New facts about disease, new drugs and instruments to treat disease, and new concepts and speculations arrive daily in a continually rising torrent. To tame the flood by understanding it we need new words to describe the new things. It is no good regretting ancient simplicities. The most we can do is to try to ensure that new words are not introduced without very good cause, and that their sense is as precise and obvious as possible. The best new words are those that are so apt and necessary that they insinuate themselves into our daily speech before we realize they are new.

Words that exactly parallel advances in knowledge make themselves. The Romans called the white of egg *albumen* (*alba*, white). The name was extended to the more or less similar protein in the blood plasma. Early last century two other proteins were separated from it, the one that gave rise to blood clots (fibrin) being naturally called *fibrinogen*; the other, resembling some vegetable proteins already so named, was called *globulin*. Biochemists divided the latter into α, β, and γ fractions without affecting language, until a sudden eruption of new knowledge about mechanisms of immunity rocketed *gamma-globulin* into (almost) a household word. In its train came by a natural process *hypergammaglobulinaemia* and *agammaglobulinaemia*, and – a singular abbreviation, leaving out the very backbone of the word – *gammopathy*, a general term for diseases involving abnormal gammaglobulin.

At the other extreme are words which represent nothing with any real existence. Blood, bile and phlegm (i.e. the nose-running of a cold, or the thick spit of bronchitis) are realities, but the four 'humours' which were conjured out of these three things and dominated medical theory for fifteen hundred years seem now the merest figments of the imagination.

More recent examples are *diathesis* and *rheumatism* (see p. 12). But we are near enough to the two latter to realize that they meant something useful to those who used them originally. Patients differ in their reactions to infections and poisons: to ascribe these differences to a diathesis may have been a mere smoke-screen to cover ignorance, but at least it tagged the phenomenon as something that existed, to be explained some day in terms of immunity and genetic differences. Even words like these have had their uses. They present, however, always the risk of the assumption that merely because they exist they must represent something. So familiar and scientific-looking a word as 'rheumatism' must mean something – but what? A general term for painful joint disease of unknown cause, a dictionary might say – but then what is muscular rheumatism?

Between the two poles of the inevitable new word that goes with major new facts and the specious coining of baseless speculation, there are all gradations. In practice, time is usually the best judge. To take a good example of a field where names often run riot, some enthusiastic group will often re-classify a group of tumours, and devise a whole set of new names to suit. If the classification proves unsound, the names will disappear (though often far too slowly). If it sticks, so probably will the names, though instead the old ones may be re-defined.

It cannot be too much emphasized that, as in evolution, the only real test of a new word is its survival. If it is a good word, its survival is more likely, but no matter how good it is, if it does not catch on regrets are useless. If it is widely used, no matter how mongrel its pedigree or vague its meaning, it has to be accepted. That does not mean one cannot do one's best to ensure the survival and proper use of good words, and to avoid propagating bad ones: only that the margin for effective action is small, and it is no use kicking against a *fait accompli*.

'GOOD' NEW NAMES. A few guidelines on what one should count as 'good' in a new word.

1. It must either stand for something newly discovered, acting as a flag for some new item of knowledge, or define something more fully and precisely than any existing word.

2. It must be clearly distinct from any existing word in

form as well as sense. Resemblance between words from widely different fields, however (even *ilium* for bone and *ileum* for intestine), matters relatively little.

3. Its sense should if possible be obvious on inspection. *Hypogammaglobulinaemia* (mouthful though it is), for example, hardly needs definition. Where this is not possible the word should at least help to jog the memory as to its meaning by some key association. *Thalassaemia* for instance means literally 'sea-blood', but the association of this particular form of anaemia with the Mediterranean is sufficient connexion (that was after all *the* sea to the Greeks – though to be sure the famous cry of 'thalassa! thalassa!', at the climax of Xenophon's tale of the retreat of the ten thousand, referred to the Black Sea).

4. It should be as short as possible and not too impossible to pronounce. As we try to use our limited stock of internationally accepted word-elements for more and more senses, this gets harder. In the case of rare diseases, a long word or a group of long words is justifiable, but length is a great nuisance with popular words (hence the plague of acronyms – see p. 99). The absence of what one would have expected to be the essential 'globulin' element from the word gammopathy (p. 36) is an example of one rather cavalier way of dealing with long words. It is not really so difficult to invent reasonably short words that carry some kind of obvious message – the drug firms do it every day, for they make a good part of their profits from attractive new names for old products.

5. It should be readily translatable into as many other languages as possible. This in practice means use as much as possible of the internationally accepted classical word-elements. (Eponyms and geographical names are fairly readily accepted overseas also.)

6. Finally, it must survive the test of actual use, and prove acceptable to today's real arbiters of elegance, the editors of our better-edited journals, and the writers of well-written monographs and textbooks. The writer of a successful student textbook has a very special respons-

ibility here: any word he uses is almost guaranteed currency during the lifetime of the students who read it.

THE VERNACULAR AND THE CLASSICAL-SCIENTIFIC. A problem often arises over choice between a good, solid Old English name and a new one. Often it is no more nor less than that constant choice in writing and speaking good English between the blunt and the decorated – truth or terminological exactitude, beauty or pulchritudinousness. Which is to say that one should use the honest kersey English when one can – gout rather than uricaemia, whooping cough rather than pertussis. There are many cases, of course, when one has no choice. Yellow fever, remarkably enough, seems never to have had any other name (except translations like *fièvre jaune*). In contrast, cholera has never had a vernacular name, and scabies has entirely ousted the old name of 'the scab' (p. 108).

There are, however, many occasions when the 'scientific' terms, jargon though they may be, have advantages. If one is writing, even in English, for an international audience – which means whenever one writes for a journal of any importance – it is as well to use as much as possible words that are readily understood by non-anglophones (jargon for those who do not speak English). Who, struggling to read a paper in German, does not curse the author who insists on writing Sauerstoff instead of oxygen, or Zwölffingerdarm for duodenum, even though the latter words would be as well understood by his countrymen as the native version?

When it comes to modifying the original words, again there are often advantages in avoiding the vernacular. It is sound practice in appropriate circumstances to say simply that the blood sugar is too low: but if you want to discuss the causes or consequences of low blood sugar in detail, you will find it far more convenient to talk of *hypoglycaemia* – sentence construction becomes far more flexible. Words like *varioliform* come easier to the tongue than smallpox-like, *maculopapular* than spotty-lumpy, and *carcinogenic* than cancer-productive. Words of unmistakable meaning such as *juxta-aortic* or *peri-thymic* can be used (or invented freely for the nonce) to replace multi-word phrases often repeated. There is no certain rule in these things: one needs tact, experience and above all attention to the kind of audience one is dealing with.

SHIFTS OF MEANING. Medical words move continuously in their sense and range of application – a few words for large anatomical structures being the only major exception. Most often this is in the direction of limitation, words being more precisely defined with time. The change of the endings *-itis* (from any disease to inflammation) and *-oma* (from any swelling to tumour) are typical. Fever no longer means any febrile disease, but only the actual fact of raised temperature; typhus no longer includes typhoid, or typhoid paratyphoid.

The reverse process is much to be deplored – the debasement of terms by over-popularity, with loss of most of their meaning. *Morbid* once meant simply diseased, in a sense for which we now often use pathological (with rather doubtful justification except need and use): its fall derived from its use in phrases like morbid fancies and morbid fears, meanings originally implying mental disease but adopted enthusiastically by novelists and the populace in the present usual sense of merely 'nasty'. *Empiric* originally meant a man who preferred facts to theories, was debased into a term of abuse for a quack doctor, and has been rehabilitated as 'empirical' into something like its original sense. *Allergy* has lost much of its value since it became a popular word for any kind of unusual reaction. *Parameter* is a particularly vicious recent example. It has a useful precise sense in mathematics, yet another in statistics and another in computing. But it began to be used for any measurable quantity (the right name for which is *variable*) among non-mathematical medical scientists, and has degenerated rapidly into a vogue-word meaning nothing at all.

The causes that a lover of the language can embrace are nearly always lost already, but the defence of good words against popular debasement ought never to be given up without a struggle.

ON BEING CLASSICALLY CORRECT

There still are, I believe, a few people who both understand the 'rules' of word-formation that Euripides and Cicero followed and believe that they ought to be applied to English words derived from Greek and Latin sources. There are others who do not understand the rules, but try to follow them all the same. And there are a multitude who neither understand nor follow the rules, but have a bad conscience about the matter. Ffrangcon Roberts in earlier editions of this book expressed a tolerant middle course, explaining the rules, and recommending their partial acceptance, but recognizing that they had long ceased to be wholly valid. The present editor takes a substantially more permissive attitude. We no longer require Latin for entry to medical school, and the background knowledge necessary to easy conformity with the old rules is lacking. To use Greek plurals for English words is now simply an affectation of knowledge we do not possess.

The rules, however, are interesting, and no one need be discouraged from using them if he wishes. They are given here together almost exactly in Ffrangcon Roberts' words:-

1. *Hybrid words*. Medical writers are frequently accused of using hybrid Greek-Latin, Greek-English and Latin-English words. Such words should be avoided if possible. For example, *phlebography* should be used instead of *venography*. But however much they may offend the purist hybrid words are often unavoidable. Even in ordinary speech they abound. In *On the Art of Writing*, by the late Sir Arthur Quiller-Couch, occurs this passage:

"I was waiting, the other day, in a doctor's anteroom, and picked up one of those books – it was a work on pathology – so thoughtfully left lying in such places; to persuade us, no doubt, to bear the ills we have rather than fly to others capable of being illustrated. I found myself engaged in following the antics of certain bacilli generically described as 'Antibodies'.... I say that for our own self-respect, whilst we retain any sense of intellectual pedigree, 'antibody' is no word to throw even at a bacillus. The man who eats peas with his knife can at least claim a historical throwback to the days when forks had but two prongs and the spoons had been removed with the soup. But 'antibody' has no such respectable derivation. It is, in fact, a barbarism, and a mongrel at that. The man who uses it debases the currency of learning."

Severe castigation indeed! Observe, however, that in the very first sentence the censorious writer himself uses *anteroom,* a mongrel word if ever there was one, half-Latin and half-Teutonic.

2. LIMITATION ON LATIN WORD FORMATION. Complicated words should be built up from Greek elements only. Latin words should be generally limited to adjectival forms and to the addition to the stem of prefixes only, except in hyphenated words such as *cerebro-spinal*. The Romans did not accept the Greek habit of joining major parts of speech together.

3. THE PLURAL. In the formation of the plural there is wide inconsistency, sometimes the grammatical forms and sometimes the anglicized form being used. It is impossible to lay down any definite rule. It is perfectly legitimate to use the anglicized form in words which have been adopted into English, and it is better to be guided by custom and euphony rather than to adhere pedantically to classical grammar. It happens that we say *corpora* and not *corpuses,* though we say *choruses* and not *chori*. Similarly we say *gladioli* and *antirrhinums*. *Stigmata* sounds better than *stigmas; carcinomas* and *carcinomata* are both correct; *enemata* is pedantic. In some words the anglicized form avoids confusion. Latin words of the fourth declension, such as *sinus,* are the same in the singular and plural; it is, therefore, essential to say *sinuses*.

4. GENDERS. It is essential to know the gender of a noun in order to make the accompanying adjective correct. Latin words ending in *us* and Greek words ending in *os* are usually masculine, while Latin words ending in *um* and Greek words ending in *on* are invariably neuter. Mistakes are most likely to arise through not knowing whether a word ending in *a* is Latin and feminine or Greek and neuter: *substantia nigra, erythema nodosum*.

The present editor believes that, even in this mild form, these rules cease to be relevant once a word or a word element has become a living part of the English language. English words, however derived, need only be subject to the rules of English grammar. The rule concerning the mixing of Greek, Latin and other word-elements has long been dead in practice, and need not be lamented. Words like speedometer and breathalyser admirably illustrate the cheerful welcome our language gives to the grossest examples of miscegenation. We were always a mixed race ourselves after all, and growing mixeder.

Plurals are the crux of the matter. Most of us religiously use the 'correct' plurals of the words familiar to us, and do our best with the rest, sometimes with confusing results – is the word *trabecula* singular (pl. *trabeculae*) or plural (sing. *trabeculum*)? It is surely better and simpler to go the whole hog, admit that the normal English -s plural (trabeculums) is *always* corect and *always* preferable. A good example is *epididymis* – must we continue to say epididymides where the English plural could be epididymises or even euphoniously and simply epididymes? We can then get rid of nonsensides like nephritides and appendicitides. Carcinomas, sulcuses, sinuses, pinnas arise! you have nothing to lose but your catenas.

We never, after all, worry about the correct plural of words from other languages. What in the original language is the plural of arpeggio, lebensraum, samovar, sampan, thug, wadi, orang-utang? Why should we kow-tow to Latin and Greek and to no living language? (and how, incidentally, would you conjugate the verb to kow-tow?).

The gender problem presented by pieces of crude Latin such as *substantia nigra*, *dermatitis herpetiformis* and *erythema nodosum* is of a different order. We learn these nowadays as semi-naturalized fossils, and only the rash or the very erudite try to handle them as genuine Latin constructions. The wary simply avoid having to make plurals by circumlocutions like 'three cases of' or 'five varieties of' erythema nodosum. Yet there is no reason to be ashamed of saying 'there are three erythema nodosums in the ward'. The truth is that such names are out of place in modern English. At least no new ones should be invented, and where ever possible they should be anglicized. '*Nodose erythema*' would be the obvious solution, were it not that the dermatologists love their *catenae*.

It is not always easy. The present editor, in spite of his principles, still finds it hard to say stratums, or naevuses, or criterions. But it comes easier with practice.

PART III

EXEMPLARY WORD LISTS

The principles which have so far been discussed are here illustrated by a large collection of Greek and Latin words with the English medical terms derived from them. They have been collected in a series of lists, based chiefly on sense (if you need to find an individual word, use the word index on p. 120). In general, when the stem which is used in English is not well shown by the nominative, the genitive case is given as well.

1. GREEK-LATIN SYNONYMS

Though Latin often borrowed Greek words for scientific purposes, in many cases both Greek and Latin originals exist, sometimes recognizably related, sometimes quite different. Often we use both, nearly always with a useful difference in exact meaning. Often the Latin word was borrowed first, and the Greek word adopted later as a basis for rather more specialized and precisely defined words. This section gives examples, all anatomical. It will be found a fascinating exercise to work out the different senses, so only a few of the more recondite variant meanings have been given in brackets.

GREEK	LATIN	ENGLISH USAGE
aden	*glans*	gland
ancone	*cubitum*	elbow (cubital fossa, anconeus muscle)
arthron	*articulatio*	joint

balanos	*glans penis*	glans penis
blepharon	*palpebra*	eyelid
cardia	*cor*, cordis	heart
cephale	*caput* (modified to *ceps* in biceps, triceps)	head
cercos	*cauda*	tail (*Cercaria* is the tailed larva of various parasitic worms)
cheilos	*labium*	lip
cheir	*manus*	hand
chondros	*cartilago*	cartilage
cleis, cleidos	*clavicula* dim. of *clavis*	clavicle (sterno-*cleido*mastoid)
cneme	*crus*	leg (gastro*cnemius*)
colpos	*vagina*	vagina
creas, creatos also **sarx, sarcos**	*caro, carnis*	flesh
cytos	*cella*	cell
dactylos	*digitus*	finger or toe
derma, dermatos also **pella**	*cutis, corium*	skin
encephalon	*cerebrum*	brain
enteron	*intestinus*	intestine
epiploon	*omentum*	omentum
epision	*pubis*	pubis
ethmoid	*cribrum*	sieve
glossa, or **glotta**	*lingua*	tongue
gnathos	*maxilla, mandibulum*	jaw
haima, haimatos	*sanguis*	blood
hystera also **metra, delphys**	*uterus*	uterus
ischion	*coxa*	hip
mastos	*mamma*	breast
myelos	*medulla*	marrow
mys, myos	*musculus*	muscle
nephros	*ren*	kidney
neuron	*nervus*	nerve
odous, odontos	*dens, dentis*	tooth

omphalos	*umbilicus*	navel
omos	*humerus*	shoulder
onyx, onychos	*unguis*	nail (*onychogryphosis*)
*****oön**	*ovum*	ovum, egg
*****oöphoron**	*ovarium*	ovary
ophthalmos	*oculus*	eye
orchis, orchidis	*testis*	testicle
organon	*viscus*	organ
osteon	*os, ossis*	bone
ous, otos	*auris*	ear
perone	*tibia*	tibia
perone	*fibula*	fibula (both words originally meant brooch-pin)
phallos	*penis*	penis
phleps, phlebos	*vena*	vein
pleumon or **pneumon**	*pulmo, pulmonis*	lung
pous, podos	*pes, pedis*	foot
proctos	*anus*	anus
pyelos	*pelvis*	pelvis
rhachis	*spina*	spine (rachitic: see p. 21)
rhis, rhinos	*nasus*	nose
soma, somatos	*corpus, corporis*	body
splanchna	*viscera*	viscera
splen	*lien*	spleen
spondylos	*vertebra*	vertebra
stethos	*thorax, thoracis*	chest
stoma	*os, oris* *bucca*	mouth
tenon	*tendo*	tendon
trachelos	*cervix, cervicis*	neck (several old trachelo- words, but none now current)

---

* In *oö*, the first *o* is long, as in *oh*, the second, short, as in *on*. Hence *oon* is pronounced *oh-on*, and *oophoron*, *oh-offeron*.

2. RESEMBLANCE

A. *Words derived with little or no alteration*

ala, L.	wing.
allantois	*allos, allantos,* sausage.
ansa, L.	handle of jug; *ansa hypoglossi.*
ascaris	roundworm.
axon	axle.
calcar, L.	spur; *calcarine, calcaneus.*
carina, L.	keel.
chiasma	two lines crossing as in the Greek letter X.
choana	funnel.
coccyx	*coccos,* cuckoo, beak of a cuckoo (sect. 10)
cochlea, L.	snail-shell.
gubernaculum, L.	helm (cf. govern).
hamus, L.	hook; *os hamatum*; dim. *hamulus,* a little hook.
haustrum, L.	an endless chain with buckets for raising water. In *haustrations* the mucosal pockets suggest the buckets.
helmin, -nthos	helminth (worm)
hilum, L.	point of attachment of a seed.
hippocampus	*hippos,* horse, *campos,* sea-monster, seahorse.
incus, L.	anvil.
infundibulum, L.	funnel.
lens, L.	lentil.
malleus, L.	hammer (cf. malleable).
manubrium, L.	handle.
pecten, L.	comb.
pinus, L.	pine-cone; *pineal.*
pinna, L.	feather.
sella, L.	saddle.
stapes, stapedis, L.	stirrup.
sustentaculum, L.	prop.
syrinx, syringos	pipe. *syringe; syringomyelia,* cavities in spinal cord.
tectorium, L.	covering, roof.
taenia	tape (worm).
tentorium, L.	tent.
tibia, L.	pipe or flute.
trochlea, *L.*	G. *trochos,* wheel, pulley.

tympanum, L., from G. *tympanon*	drum.
umbilicus, L.	dim. of *umbo*, boss on a shield.
vomer. L.	ploughshare.

B. *By the addition, originally only to Greek words, of* oid, *"in the form of"* (G. eidos, *form*)

adenoid	*aden*, gland, i.e. a gland-like mass that is not a gland.
arachnoid	*arachne*, spider's web.
arytaenoid	*arytainos*, cup or ladle.
choroid	*chorion*, leather or parchment.
cirsoid	*cirsos*, varix.
clinoid	*cline*, bed. The clinoid processes resembles the posts of a four-poster bed, the *diaphragma sellae* being the canopy.
colloid	*colla*, glue.
coracoid	*corax, coraces*, crow, beak of a crow. See section 10.
coronoid	*corone*, crow, beak of a crow. See section 10.
cricoid	*cricos*, ring.
cuboid	*cubos*, cube.
deltoid	G. letter *delta*, Δ, hence triangular.
desmoid	*desmos*, band, ligaments.
ethmoid	*ethmos*, sieve.
fibroid	*fibra*, L., thread, i.e. like fibrous tissue.
glenoid	*glene*, shallow socket.
hyoid	G. letter *upsilon*, i.e. U-shaped.
lambdoid	G. letter *lambda*, λ.
lipoid	*lipos*, fat.
mastoid	*mastos*, breast.
odontoid	*odous, odontos*, tooth.
pterygoid	*pteryx, pterygos*, wing.
scaphoid	*scaphe*, boat.
sesamoid	*sesame*, seed.
sigmoid	G. letter *sigma*, i.e. S-shaped.
sphenoid	*sphen*, wedge.
styloid	*stylos*, pillar.
thyroid	*thyreos*, shield. This was the long shield, on the upper edge of which was a notch for the wearer's chin. The e is occasionally seen, and

was for a time official in the BNA anatomy nomenclature, but though strictly correct it is now an affectation (i.e. *thyreoid*).

trapezoid	*trapezion*, small table.
typhoid	*typhos*, smoke or mist (p. 17).
xiphoid	*xiphos*, sword.

C. *By the addition, generally to Latin words, of* iform

cribriform	*cribrum*, sieve.
cuneiform	*cuneus*, wedge.
ensiform	*ensis*, sword.
falciform	*falx, falcis*, scythe.
fungiform	*fungus*, mushroom.
fusiform	*fusus*, spindle.
mammilliform	*mammilla*, dim. of *mamma*, breast.
pampiniform	*pampinus*, tendril.
pisiform	*pisum*, pea.
pyriform	*pirus*, pear.
restiform	*restis*, rope.
unciform	*uncus*, hook.

D. *By the prefix* pseudo (pseudo, *false*) *which often carries an overtone of deception.*

pseudocyesis	false pregnancy.
pseudoleukaemia	apparent leukaemia.
pseudomembranous	imitating membranous (inflammation).

3. DIMINUTIVES

A. *In Latin words by inserting between the stem and the ending of the letter* l, *alone or in combination—ol, iol, ell, scl, ul, cul.*

areola	area.
auricle	*auris*, ear.
bacillus	*baculus*, rod.
bronchiole	*bronchus*.
calculus	*calx*, pebble.
capitellum	*caput*, head.

capsule	*capsa*, box.
caruncle	*caro*, flesh
cerebellum	*cerebrum*.
corpuscle	*corpus*, body.
diverticulum	*diversum*, diversion.
flagellum	*flagrum*, scourge.
flocculus	*flocus*, tuft of wool.
follicle	*follis*, bag.
fontanelle	*fontana*, fountain (p. 14).
frenulum	*frenum*, bridle.
globulin	*globus*, ball.
habenula	*habena*, bridle-rein.
hamulus	*hamus*, hook.
lingula	*lingua*, tongue.
lobule	*lobus*, lobe.
malleolus	*malleus*, hammer.
morula	*morus*, mulberry.
navicular	*navis*, ship.
nodule	*nodus*, knob.
nucleolus	(double diminutive) lit. very small nut.
nucleus	*nux*, nut.
ossicle	*os, ossis*, bone.
pedicle **pediculus** **peduncle**	*pes, pedis*, foot.
saccule	*saccus*, bag.
tubercle	*tuber*, swelling.
umbilicus	*umbo*, shield.
utricle	*uterus*.
uvula	*uva*, bunch of grapes.
vascular	*vas*, vessel.
ventricle	*venter*, belly.
vesicular	*vesica*, bladder.

B. *In Greek words by the insertion of* e, i *or* ei *after the stem, the ending remaining or becoming neuter:*

angeion	*angon*, box: angioma, angiography, haemangioma, etc.
bacterium	L. from G. *bacterion*, dim. of *bactron*, rod.
chondrion	*chondros*, cartilage or granule: mitochrondria, lit. granular threads.

histion　　　*histos*, tissue: histiocyte, wandering cell of connective tissue.

C. *By the addition of* idium, *the latinized form of G.* idion *to the stem:*

clostridium　　　*closter*, spindle.
coccidium　　　*coccus*, berry.
oidium　　　*oon*, ovum, egg.

4. RECEPTACLES, CAVITIES

alveolus, L.	small cavity dim. of *alveus*.	alveoli of the lung; alveolar process of mandible because it holds sockets for teeth.
amphoreus	jar	amphoric
ampulla, L.	flask	ampulla of Vater.
antron	cave	maxillary antrum.
ascos	bag	ascites, the abdomen resembling a bag.
atrium, L.	room	syn. auricle.
bothrios	small pit	bothriocephalus (the fish tapeworm).
bursa, L.	purse (cf. bursar, one who keeps the purse).	
calyx, calycis, L.	cup	
caverna, L.	cavern	cavernous sinus.
cella, L.	chamber	cell.
cestos	belt	cestode (tapeworm).
cisterna, L.	reservoir	
coilia	belly	coeliac, coelom.
cystis	bladder	cyst, cystitis, etc.
dochos	container	choledochos, gallbladder.
folliculus, L.	small bag, dim. of *follis*.	follicle, follicular.

EXEMPLARY WORD LISTS

fovea, L.	pit, depression	fovea centralis of retina.
gaster	stomach, belly	gastric, epigastric, etc.

Note.—*Gaster*, like *belly*, is used to indicate protuberance as well as cavity. It depends whether one looks at the outside or the inside; e.g. digastric muscle, muscle with two swellings or bellies; gastrocnemius, i.e. swelling of leg (*cneme*. leg).

involucrum, L.	envelope	
lacuna, L.	pool, hollow	
patella, L.	small dish, pan, dim of *patina*.	
pelvis, L.	basin	
pyelos	basin	pyelitis.
sacculus, L.	small bag, dim. of *saccus*	saccule of ear.
sinus, L.	hollow, curve	(cf. E. sine, sinuous); nasal sinuses; venous channels in the dura mater; artificial and pathological openings to the surface.
stria, L.	furrow	striated.
stroma	bed, covering	
sulcus, L.	furrow	
tectum, tegmentum, L.	covering	tectorium, tegmen tympani, integument.
theca	receptacle	
tunica	a covering	tunica albuginea (cf. tunic).
vagina, L.	sheath	
vas, L.	vessel	dim. adj. vascular.
venter, L.	belly	used only as adj. ventral and dim. ventricle.
vestibulum, L.	vestibule	vestibular nerve, vestibule of internal ear.
vulva, L.	wrapper	

5. MEMBRANES AND PARTITIONS

chorion	leather, parchment, skin.	
hymen	originally any membrane.	
mediastinum, L.	lit. something standing between, a common servant (cf. 'tweeny').	
membrana, L.	membrane.	
meninx, mening-	membrane, esp. of brain	meninges.
paries, parietis, L.	wall	parietal.
phragma	wall	diaphragm.
septum, L.	partition.	

6. OPENINGS AND COMMUNICATIONS

aditus, L.	approach to	aditus ad antrum.
ductus, L.	duct	ductus arteriosus, aqueduct.
fenestra, L.	window	fenestra ovalis.
fistula, L.	pipe	
foramen, L. pl. **foramina**	hole	
hiatus, L.	opening or space	
iter, L.	journey	passage between third and fourth ventricles. ventricles.
meatus, L.	channel	
operculum, L.	lid	
os, oris, L.	mouth	oral.
ostium, L.	opening	ostium abdominale.
patulus, L.	standing open	patulous.
poros	passage, pore	porous.
rima, L.	slit	rima glottidis.
sinus, L.	fold, bay	
spadion	tear, rent	epispadias, hypospadias (abnormal openings of the urethra.
stoma, stomatos	mouth	stomach, stomatitis; anastomosis, a communication between vessels or cavities of organs.

trema	hole	helicotrema.
tresis	hole	atresia, congenital imperforation as in the anus or the lower end of the oesophagus.

7. TEXTURE, FABRICS

arachne	spider's web	arachnoid mater
cancellus, L.	lattice-work	cancellous tissue of bone.
diphthera	parchment	diphtheria (from membrane in throat).
endyma	garment	ependyma.
fascia, L.	band or bundle	
fasciculus, L.	dim. of fascia	fascicular.
fibra, L.	thread	fibre, fibrous tissue, etc.
filum, L.	thread	filaria, filiform.
fimbria, L.	fibre	fimbriated.
flocculus, L.	tuft of wool	flocculated.
ganglion	knot	hence swelling like a knot on a nerve and on back of wrist.
glomus, L.	skein of wool	dim. glomerulus.
histos	tissue, originally loom	histology, etc.
lemniscus, L.	band or fillet	
limbus, L.	border	
mitos	thread	mitosis, lit. a state of being in threads, the state of the chromatin bodies in cell-division.
nema, nematos	thread	nematode, i.e. worm like a thread.
pannus, L.	garment	dim. *panniculus*.
plexus, L.	woven	complex.
plica, L,	fold	complicated, etc.
pulvinar, L.	pillow	posterior tubercle of thalamus.

rete, L.	net	
reticulum, L.	fine net	reticulated.
ruga, L.	crease	
spongos	sponge	spongioblast, primitive neurological cell.
tainia (taenia, L.)	tape, ribbon	taenia, tapeworm.
tapes, tapetos	carpet	tapetum (cf. tapestry).

8. AIR, BREATH

aer	air	aerophagy (eating air); anaerobic.
aither	ether	upper air.
asthma	panting	
atmos	air, stream	atmosphere.
aura, L.	breeze	meaning transferred to the sensations which precede an epileptic fit..
capnos	smoke	acapnia, deficiency of CO_2, in blood, CO_2 being figuratively as smoke.
halitus, L.	vapour	halitosis (p. 17).
pneuma	air, spirit	pneumonia, pneumogastric, etc. (p. 11).
pnoe	breathing	apnoea, dyspnoea, orthopnoea (see section 17).
zoe	life	azotaemia, via F. *azote*, nitrogen.

9. FLUIDS

bilis, L.	bile	urobilin.
chole	bile	cholecystitis, cholera (p. 11).
haima	blood	haemorrhage (p. 11).
sanguis, sanguinis, L.		sanguineous, sanguine.
chylos	juice	Usually restricted to the fat-containing lymph which passes along the lacteals from the intestine, though in *achylia gastrica* it refers to gastric juice.

chymos	juice	Food in process of digestion; parenchyma (p. 19) (ecchymosis is a misnomer for echaemosis).
lympha, L.	clear water	lymphocytes, etc.
lac, lactis, L.	milk	lacteals, lactic acid, etc.
gala, galactos	milk	galactose, sugar present in milk; galactogogue (sect. 33); galactocele.
mucus, L.	(nasal) mucus	mucin, mucous glands, etc.
myxa	slime	myxoedema, myxoma.
blennos	slime	blennorrhoea.
plasma	plasma	lit. anything formed (p. 84): the fluid part of the blood, presumably from its ability to form a clot.
pyon	pus	pyo-, suppurate, empyema, pyaemia, etc.
sialon	saliva	sialography.
serum, L.	whey	the fluid exuding from a blood-clot.
hidros	sweat	hyperhidrosis; hidradenoma.
sudor, L.	sweat	sudorific glands
lacrima, L.	tear	lacrimal or (a mediaeval decoration) lachrymal gland.
dacryon	tear	dacryocystitis (inflammation of lacrimal gland).
ouron, urina, L.	urine	urea, ureter, urethra, diuresis (lit. urine passing through).
aqua, L.	water	
hydor, hydro-	water	
copros	faeces	
faex, faecis, L.	dregs	
scybalon	dung	used in pl. *scybala*.

stercus, L.	dung	stercobilin; stercorous, having a faecal smell.

10. ANIMALS

zoon		zoology.
entoma	insect	entomology.
pediculus, L.	louse	
pulex, L.	flea	
bous	ox	buphthalmos.
canis, L.	dog	canine teeth.
carcinoma,	crab	malignant tumour (p. 104).
cancer, L.	crab	
coccos	cuckoo	
corax, coracos	crow	
corone	crow	

The Greeks also used these words for the birds' curved beaks and for hooked or curved objects, such as door-handles, which resemble beaks. Hence coccyx, coracoid and coronoid. *Corone* also meant wreath, garland or similar circular object. Hence in the latinized form, *corona,* we have coronal suture, the suture where the garland is placed (cf, crown), and coronary arteries, arteries which surround the heart.

elephas, elephantis	elephant	elephantiasis.
equus, L.	horse	equinovarus; cauda equina.
hippos	horse	hippocampus (sect. 2).

lagos	hare	lagophthalmos, inability to close the eyes.
leo, leontis, L.	lion	leontiasis.
lumbricus, L.	worm	lumbrical muscles.
lupus, L.	wolf	lupus, something which devours.
mys, myos	mouse	also means muscle. The synonym may have arisen through muscles suggesting mice under the skin. Cf. lumbricals.
musca, L.	fly	muscae volitantes (lit. flying flies).
phryne	frog	phrynoderma.
rana, L.	frog	ranula.
psittacos	parrot	psittacosis.
rhesus	(name of a king of Thrace)	monkey concerned in blood grouping

11. PLANTS

phyton	plant	saprophyte (sect. 46); epidermophyton, lit. plant growing on the epidermis.
coccos	berry	staphylococcus, etc.
karyon	nut	hence nucleus; megakaryocyte, cell with large nucleus; karyokinesis, lit. movement of nucleus, syn. mitosis.
leichen	moss	lichen.
lens, L.	lentil	lens, from the shape; lentiform.
phakos	lentil	hence lens; aphakia, absence of lens; phacoscope.
mekon	poppy	meconium, the infant's first anal excretion, from the resemblance to poppy-seed oil.
milium, L.	millet seed	miliary tuberculosis.
myces	fungus	mycology; actinomycosis, infection with ray fungus (*actis, actinis,* ray); antibiotics derived from

		fungi—streptomycin, terramycin, aureomycin, etc.
nux, L.	nut	hence nucleus, used in dim. nucleus, nucleolus (sect. 3).
sycon	fig	sycosis, from a supposed resemblance.
urtica, L.	nettle	urticaria, nettle-rash.
uva, L.	grape	uvea, uvula.
zyme	yeast	enzyme, zymotic.

12. SUBSTANCES

acetum, L.	vinegar	acetabulum (vinegar cup).
adeps, adipis, L.	fat	adipose.
albumen, L.	white of egg	albuginea.
amylon	starch	amylase, amyloid disease.
anthrax, anthracis	coal	anthrax (p. 16).
byssos	flax, cotton	byssinosis.
calx, calcis, L.	chalk	calcareous, calcification.
carbo, carbonis, L.	coal	carbuncle (p. 16).
caseus, L.	cheese	caseous, casein.
colla	glue	colloid, collagen.
conis	dust	pneumoconiosis.
electron	amber	electrode, etc.
farina	starch	farinaceous
glia	glue	neuroglia, i.e. binding cells; glioma.
glus, glutis, L.	glue	agglutination.
kalium (p. 95)	potassium	kaliuresis, excess of potassium in urine.
lecithos	yolk of egg	lecithin.
lipos	fat	lipase, lipoma.
lithos	stone	lithotomy, cutting for removal of stone.
natrium (p. 95)	sodium	natriuresis, excess of sodium in urine.
psammos	sand	psammoma, brain tumour containing gritty particles.
sebum, L.	tallow	sebaceous, seborrhoea.

sideros	iron	siderosis.
smegma	grease	
stear, steatos	fat	stearic, steatorrhoea.
synovia, L.	white of egg	synovial fluid.
vitellus, L.	yolk of egg	vitelline duct.
xylon	wood	haematoxylin.

13. QUANTITY, DEFICIENCY, EXCESS

pan total panhysterectomy, pancreas (all flesh).
plethora fullness.

Deficiency
1. The alpha privative, **a,** before a consonant, **an,** before a vowel or *h*. This expresses either complete absence, as in achlorhydria, anencephalic, or relative deficiency as in anaemia. The alpha privative is not to be confused with *ana,* up, back.
2. **pen,** from *penia,* thrombocytopenia, deficiency of clot-forming cells; leuco(cyto) penia, defiiency of white cells (p. 116).
lack
3. **oligos** few oligospermia; oligodendroglia, cells of the neuroglia with few branches.
4. **in, im,** L. not imbalance (cf. impatient).
5. **hypo** under hypotonic, hypochromic, etc.

Excess
1. **hyper** hyperaemia, hyperglycaemia, hypertrophy.
2. **poly** polycythaemia (too) many blood cells; poly also means many (apart from too many); polypus, lit. many-feet; polymorphonuclear. L. equivalent, *multus,* multilocular.

More **pleion** (combining form pleo) pleomorphic, having more than one form.

14. NUMBERS
(combining forms)

		GREEK	LATIN
CARDINAL	one	**mono-**	*un-*
	two	**di-**	*bi-*
	three	**tri-**	*ter-*
	four	**tetr-**	*quadr-*
	five	**pent-**	*quinqu-*
	six	**hex-**	*sex-*
	seven	**hept-**	*sept-*
	eight	**oct-**	*oct-*
	nine	**ennea-**	*novem-*
	ten	**dec-**	*decem-*
	hundred	**hect-**	*cent-*
	thousand	**kilo-**	*milli-*
	half	**hemi-**	*semi-*
ORDINAL	first	**prot-**	*prim-*
	second	**deuter-**	*secund-*
	third	**trit-**	*tert-*

15. PAIRED AND UNPAIRED

ambo, L.	both	amboceptor; ambidextrous.
ampi	both	amphibian.
di-	two	dicrotic, double beat; uterus didelphys, double uterus. diplegia, paralysis of both legs; distomum hepaticum, liver fluke, digastric, double-bellied (muscle).
didymi	twins	epididymis, the twins being the testes.
diplo-	double	diplopia, double vision. diplococci, cocci occurring in pairs; (in sense of between) diploe, cancellous tissue between outer and inner tables of skull.
gemini, L.	twins	bigeminal. Also trigeminal, in the sense of three parts. Corpora quadrigemina, four parts.

hapos	single	haploid, having a single set of chromosomes, as in germ cells.
monas	single	trichomonas, single-haired.
quadr-	four	corpora quadrigemina.
jugum, L.	yoke	jugular.
zygon	yoke	zygote, the cell resulting from sexual reproduction; homozygous, inheriting similar genes from the two parents; heterozygous, resulting from cross-breeding of pure but different strains; zygoma, the bone yoking the malar and temporal; azygos (unpaired) vein.

16. MEASUREMENT AND SIZE

metron	measure	emmetropic, ametropic and hypermetropic respectively, normal, defective and excessive size of the eye.
megas, megalos	large	megacolon, megaloblast.
macros		macrocyte.
magnus, L. comp. **major**; sup. **maximus**		
micros	small	microcyte.
parvus, L. comp. **minor**; sup. **minimus**		

Comparative Size

iso-	equal	isometric, isotonic.
aniso-	unequal	anisocytosis, cells of unequal size.
poikilo-	,,	poikilocytosis.

17. FORM, SHAPE

morphe	form	morphia (p. 23); morphology; polymorphonuclear, etc.
dolichos	long	dolichocephalic.
longus, L.		
brachys	short	brachycephalic, brachydactyly.

brevis, L.		cf. brief.
anus, L.	round, circular, spherical.	Now limited to one round hole, though no such restriction applies to the dim. annulus.
cyclos		cyclitis, inflammation of ciliary body; (cf. bicycle).
globus, L.		globin.
gyros		gyrus of brain; (cf. gyrate).
orbis, L.		orbicular.
rotundus, L.		foramen rotundum.
strongylos		strongyloides (worm).
teres, L.		ligamentum teres.
pessos	pebble-shaped	pessary.
eurys	wide	aneurysm, lit. a widening up.
latus, L.		latissimus (widest).
stenos	narrow	stenosis.
orthos	straight, upright	orthopaedics (p. 109); orthopnoea, ability to breathe only in upright position; also used to express normality, as in orthodox, orthochromic.
rectus, L.		rectum.
ankylos	bent	ankylosis; (cf. ankle, angle), ankylostomum.
kyphos		kyphosis, forward curvature.
scolios		scoliosis, lateral curvature.
lordos	bent backwards	lordosis.
opisthen	backwards	opisthotonus, spasm of muscles of back.
luna, L.	crescent	os lunatum.
meniscos		lit. small moon; meniscus.
oxys	sharp-pointed	amphioxus (animal pointed at both ends), oxyuris (sharp-tailed worm).
		oxys also means sharp, bitter and sudden (sects 38 and 30).
eileos	twisted	ileum, ileus.
tortus, L.		torticollis.
volvulus, L.	rolled up	

lamella, L.	flat	thin plate.
lamina, L.		thin plate; laminated.
platys	wide	platysma.
plax, placos		leucoplakia; placenta, lit. flat cake.
trigonon	triangle	trigone of bladder.
triquetrus, L.		triquetrum.
astron	star	astrocyte.
stella, L.		stellate ganglion.
cavus, L.	hollow	vena cava, because found collapsed after death.
koilos		koilonychia, lit. hollow nails.
helix	spiral	helicotrema.
speira		spirochaete, *chaite,* hair.
trepanon	gimlet	trepan, old form of trephine; trypanosome, body shaped like a gimlet; treponema.
turbo, L.	whirl	turbinate (cf. turbine).
nummus, L.	coin	nummular sputum.
monile, L.	beaded	moniliasis, moniliform.
rhabdos, rod	striated	rhabdomyoma, tumour of striated muscle.
scalenos	irregular	scalene muscles.

18. COLOUR

chroma, chromatos	colour	chromaffin, chromophil, chromophobe (sect. 37), c h r o m a t o l y s i s, chromosome.
erythros	red	erythrocyte, erythema, erysipelas (*pella,* skin).
ruber, L.		rubella (German measles), rubeola (measles), rubrospinal tract (from the red nucleus).
eos (dawn)	pink, rosy	eosin, eosinophil.
rhodon (a rose)		rhodopsin.
roseus, L.		acne rosacea.
cirros	tawny or reddish-yellow	cirrhosis (from the colour of the liver).
aureus, L.	golden	*Staphylococcus aureus.*

flavus, L.	yellow	riboflavin, ligamentum flavum.
galbus, L.		jaundice (through F. *jaune*).
icteros		icterus (jaundice).
luteus, L.		corpus luteum.
xanthos	xanthoma	
chloros	green	chlorine, chlorosis, chlorophyll.
glaucos	greyish-green	glaucoma.
cyanos	blue	cyanosis.
porphyra	purple	haematoporphyrin.
purpurus, L.		purpura.
albus, L.	white	albino, albicans, albumen, linea alba.
leucos		leucocyte, leucorrhoea, leucoderma, leucoplakia, leucocytosis, etc.
argentum, L.	silver	argentaffin cells.
argyros		hydrargyrum, mercury, lit. silver water; argyria, silver poisoning.
pallidus, L.	pale	globus pallidus, *Spirochaeta pallida*.
polios	grey	poliomyelitis, inflammation of grey matter.
ater, L.	black	atrabilious, atrium (p. 13).
melas, melanos		melanin, melanoma, melaena (p. 15).
niger, L.		substantia nigra.
amauros	dark	amaurosis, amaurotic idiocy.
scotomos	dark, gloomy	scotoma (of retina).
amblys	dull	amblyopia.
phaeos	dusky	phaechromocytoma, lit. tumour of dark-coloured cells.
iris, iridis	rainbow	

19. HARDNESS, SOFTNESS, THICKNESS, THINNESS, WEIGHT

adamas, adamantos very hard, unbreakable   adamantinoma.

callus, L., originally applied to skin	hard	callus, callosity, corpus callosum (cf. callous).
durus, L.		dura mater, indurated.
eburneus, L., lit. of ivory		eburnation (of bone in osteoarthritis).
petros		petrous bone.
scirrhos		scirrhous carcinoma.
scleros		sclera, sclerotic, sclerosis.
krauros	brittle	kraurosis vulvae.
stereos	solid	cholesterol, lit. solid substance of bile; stereognosis, ability to recognize three-dimensional shape.
malacos	soft	osteomalacia.
mollis, L.		emollient.
molluscus, L.	softish	molluscum contagiosum.
pachys	thick	pachymeningitis (affecting the dura).
spissus, L.		inspissated.
leptos	thin	leptomeningitis (affecting the pia and arachnoid).
manos		manometer. See *sphygmo* (sect. 30).
barus	heavy	barium; hyperbaric.

20. SURFACE

ichthys	fish	ichthyosis } i.e. scaly.
lepra		leprosy
squama	scale	squamous, desquamate.
keras, keratos	horn	keratin, keratitis (the cornea is of course not made of horn, but translucent horn was once used for small windows).
corneus, L.		cornea, stratum corneum.
hirsutus, L.	shaggy	hirsute.

acanthos	thorn	acanthosis.
echinos	hedgehog	echinococcus.
trachys	rough	trachea (once called the 'rough artery'); trachoma.
ruga, L.	wrinkle	rugose.
leios	smooth	leiomyoma, tumour of smooth muscle; lienteric (lit. smooth intestine).
alopex (fox)	bald	alopecia (p. 16).
siccus, L.	dry	desiccated.
skeletos		skeleton.
xeros		xeroderma.
pityron (bran)	scurfy	pityriasis.
favus, L.	honeycomb	ring-worm.
phryne (frog)	like frog's skin	phrynoderma.
bulla, pl. **bullae**, L.	blister	
pemphis		pemphigus.
phlyctaina		phlyctenular keratitis.
pompholyx		cheiropompholyx.
acne	pustule	prob. *akme*, point.
comedo, L. pl. **comedos** or **comedones**		lit. a glutton, L. *comedere*, to devour.
furunculus, L.	boil	furunculosis.
papula, L. dim. **papilla**	pimple	papular eruption.
varius, L.	spotted	variola, small-pox; varicella, chicken-pox.
ulcus, L.	ulcer	
aphtha	thrush (disease, not bird) probably	aphthous stomatitis.
dainou	eating	phagedaena, spreading ulcer, *phago-*, eat.
rhagas, pl. **rhagades**	fissure	

cicatrix, cicatricis, L.	scar	
verruca, L.	wart	
naevus, L.	wart or mole	
phyma		rhinophyma.
capillus, L.	hair	capillary.
chaite		spirochaete.
pilus, L.		pilomotor.
thrix, trichos		streptothrix, trichophyton, leptothrix.
villus, L.		
cilia, L.	eyelashes	originally in Latin the eyelid. The sing. is *cilium*.
boubon	bubo	

21. IDENTITY

autos	self	autogenous, arising within itself; autonomic (*nomos*, law), lit. a law to itself, i.e. not under the control of the will. Autism (adj. autistic) cf. automatic, automobile.
idios	individual, one's own, peculiar to oneself (p. 16).	idiopathic, lit. peculiar to or caused by itself, i.e. not by any known external cause; idiosyncrasy (*syncrasia*, temperament).
proprius, L.	one's own	proprioceptive sensations, those received from within oneself. Ant. exteroceptive.
homo, homoeo	same, like	homolateral, same side: homologous, corresponding; homoeopathy (literally 'sympathy' – p. 105); homograft, from another of the same species.

ipse	same, like	ipsilateral, syn. homolateral.
anomalos	uneven	anomaly.
heteros	other, different	heterolateral, opposite side.
contra, L.	opposite	contralateral, opposite side.
allos	other	allergy (*ergon*, work), a reaction other than the usual one.
allelon	of one another	allelomorph, one of the forms (originally thought always to occur in pairs) in which a gene expresses itself.
adventitius, L.	foreign	adventitia.

22. HUMAN RELATIONS AND AGE

demos	people	endemic, epidemic, pandemic.
ephebos	young man	ephebiatrics, medicine as applied to young men.
genos	family, race	genetics; miscegenation, mixed breeding (*miscere*, L. mix).
gamos	marriage	gamete, mature reproductive cell, egg or sperm.
gametes	husband	
gamete	wife	
atavus, L.	remote ancestor	atavism, inheritance from an ancestral type.
homo, L.	man (species)	
anthropos	man (species)	anthropoid.
aner, andros	man (sex)	androgen.
gyne, gynaecos	woman	gynaecology.
pais, paidos, dim. **paidion**	1. child of either sex 2. boy	paediatrics; orthopaedics; paederasty (*erastes*, love).
puer, L.	child	puerperium (parere, to bear).
puber, L.	adult	

pubes, L.	signs of manhood	puberty.
hebe	youth	hebephrenia (adolescent schizophrenia (sect. 26. (Not to be confused with *hebes,* dull).
parthenos	virgin	parthenogenesis.
geron	old man	geriatrics, syn. gerontology.
presbys	old man	presbyopia; presbycousis (or -acusis), deafness of old age.
senex, L.	old man	senescence.
nymphe	maiden	nymphomania.
oikos	house	ecology, study of the effects of the environment.
ontos	a being	ontogenesis, the evolution of the individual.
phylon	tribe	phylogenesis, the evolution of the race.

23. POSITION

acron	point, end, summit	acromion, point of shoulder (*omos,* shoulder); acromegaly (enlargement of extremities).
veru, L.	ridge	verumontanum.
caecus, L.	blind	caecum, blind (end).
cuspis	point, spear, sting of bee	bicuspid, tricuspid.
decubitus, L.	lying down	orig. with elbow (cubitum) on a cushion. From *decumbo,* lie down (cf. recumbent).
locus, L.	place	locomotor, lit. moving place, localization.
macula, L.	small spot	
situs, L.	site	situs inversus.

stasis, G.	standing, stopping, arrest	haemostasis; interstitial (placed between); hypostatic; statistics.
status, L.	position	lit. standing under, originally sediment; prostate, standing before (the bladder); obstetrics, L. *obstetrix, icis,* midwife lit. one who stands in front of (*ob,* in front of).
stigma	point	astigmatism (no point of focus).
stole	place, from *stellein*	systole, diastole (sect. 32).
taxis	arrangement, from *tassein,* to arrange	ataxia, lit. disarranged.
telos	end	telangiectasis, dilatation of ends of vessels.
thesis	a placing	hypothesis, lit. a placing below; diathesis, lit. a placing apart; prosthesis, an addition, fitting of artificial parts.
thetos	fixed	athetotic, unfixed, disordered.
topos	place	ectopic, out of place; ectopic gestation; ectopia vesicae; topography.

24. RELATIVE POSITION

Most of the words that belong here are used chiefly as prefixes and will be found on p. 27.

Cortex, Medulla and Myelin

In organs such as long bones and the suprarenal glands which have outer and inner parts differing in function the outer part is called the cortex (L. *bark*) and the inner part the medulla (from L. *medius,* middle), terms used for the corresponding parts in plants. The old name spleno-medullary leukaemia indicates that the spleen and the medulla (or marrow) of long bones are involved. In medullated (or white) peripheral nerve-fibres the term medulla is applied to the fatty sheath which lies between the axon or central layer and the neurilemma (Gr. *lemma,* bark).

In the central nervous system these terms are modified. The cortex is the outer part of the cerebrum and cerebellum while the medulla is the brain-stem lying between the pons and the spinal cord. Formerly it must have been used for the whole spinal cord (which could be thought of as a kind of marrow to the vertebral column), a usage which survives in *transverse myelitis* and *poliomyelitis.*

Myelin (G. myelos) is the substance of which the fatty sheath of peripheral nerve-fibres are composed. In nerve-fibres the term myelinated is syn. with medullated. Among diseases of the central nervous system we have transverse myelitis and poliomyelitis. Myeloma means tumour of (bone) marrow. Myelogenous leukaemia is syn. with spleno-medullary leukaemia.

25. ARRANGEMENT, DISTRIBUTION

acinus, L.	grape, or bunch	acini of lungs.
bothryos	of grapes	bothryomyces.
racemos		racemous glands.
staphylos		staphylococcus (*coccos,* berry); staphyloma.
uvula, L.		
arbor, L.	tree	arborisation.
dendron		dendrite, branching termination of a nerve cell.
ramus, L.	branch	ramify.
streptos	chain	streptococcus.
fascia, L.	compact	bundle.
pycnos		pyknosis, nuclei shrunken.
syncytium		lit. cells together, a mass of nuclei with no cell-divisions.
cingulum, L.	girdle	shingles.
zoster		herpes zoster.
kestus		cestode.
kremathra	hanging basket	cremaster, by which the testes are suspended

26. APPROXIMATION, SEPARATION

sy-, sym-, syn- together   systole (sect. 23); symphysis,

		lit. growing together; synostosis, lit. bones together; synapse, contact; synechiae (pl.), adhesions (*synechein*, hold together).
conjugare, L.	to unite	conjunctiva, uniting the lids with the eyeball.
petere, L.	to seek	centripetal, syn. afferent.
coitus, L.	going together	
desis	binding	arthrodesis.
desmos		syndesmosis, fibrous joint; desmoid, fibrous tumour.
ligare, L.	to bind	ligature, ligament
haptein	to touch	hapten.
pagos	fixed	craniopagus, twins attached by the head.
pexis	fastening	nephropexy.
nectere, L.	fasten together	adnexa.
rhaphe	seam	perineorrhaphy.
sphincter	binding	sphincter.
valgus, L.	bow-legged	*genu valgum*, knock-kneed (p. 20).
crinein	to separate	adopted with the sense secrete, as in endocrine.
dia-	apart	diastole (sect. 23.
fugere, L.	flee	centrifugal, syn. efferent.
schizein	split	schizophrenia; schizomycetes.
varus, L.	apart	*genu varum*, bow-legged.

27. VISIBILITY

hyalon	glass	hyaline; hyaluronidase.
lucidus, L.	transparent	stratum lucidum.
saphenes	plain	saphenous vein, because plain to see.
vitrum, L.	glass	vitreous humour.
cryptos	concealed	cryptorchidism.
occultus, L.		occult blood.

28. TEMPERATURE

therme	heat	thermometer, etc.
calor, L.	heat	calorimeter, etc.
pyr, pyros	fire	pyrexia; pyrosis, heartburn.
pyreticos	relating to fire	antipyretic, drug which subdues fever.
causis	a burning, from *causein*, to burn	causalgia, burning pain.
causticos	capable of, or related to, burning	caustic.
cauterion	branding iron	cautery.
febris, L.	fever	febrile.
fovimentum, L.	warm application	fomentation.
zeein	to boil	eczema; coryza (p. 12).
psychros	cold	psychrotherapy, treatment by application of cold.
kryos	frost	cryotherapy; cryostat.

29. TIME

chronos	time	chronic, etc.
mene	month	amenorrhoea, menorrhagia, menopause, etc.
menis, L.	month	menses.
menstruus, L.	monthly	menstrual.
luna, L.	moon, hence month	lunatic.
dies, L.	day	quotidian, daily, (*quo* as many); circadian, approximately daily (of rhythms).
nyx, nyctos	night	nyctalopia (p. 20).
nox, noctis, L.	night	nocturnal.
fugax, L.	temporary	proctalgia fugax.
praecox, L.	lit. before cooking (*pre*, before, *coquere*, L. to cook)	precocity; dementia praecox.

30. SPEED

tachys	rapid	tachycardia.
acutus, L.	sharp	acute.
oxys (sects 17 and 38)	sharp	paroxysm.
bradys	slow	bradycardia.
rhythmos	rhythm	arrhythmia.
crotos	beat	dicrotic.
diadocho-	in orderly succession or alternation	dysdiadochokinesis, difficulty in performing alternating movements.
sphyxis	pulse	asphyxia, which originally meant failure of the pulse; sphygmomanometer.

31. TENSION, RELAXATION

The root word for tension is G. **teino,** I stretch, from which there are many derivatives: G. *tonos, tetanos;* L. *tonus* and *tendere*. These have a wide use: tendon; tensor and extensor in muscle; tonus, with its derivatives atonia, hypertonic, hypotonic, catatonia; peritoneum (something stretched around); tenesmus (straining in defaecation). Note the difference between tetanus and tetany: tetanus is the disease known as lock-jaw and also the sustained contraction of muscle produced by rapid stimulation; tetany is the abnormal sensitivity of muscle produced by low calcium levels.

dynamis	power	dynamics.
piesis	pressure	hyperpiesis.
rigor, L.	stiffness (cf. rigorous)	
spasmos	spasm, convulsion.	
spasticos	drawn out, stretched, hence tight	spastic.
sthenos	strong	asthenia, weakness; neurasthenia.
tasis	stretching	myotasis; myotatic contractions.

paresis slackening, hence weakness

32. EXPANSION, CONTRACTION

chalasis	relaxation	achalasia, failure to relax.
diastole	a placing apart (*dia*, apart, *-tole*, place)	a placing apart of heart walls, i.e. dilatation.
ectasis	a stretching out	bronchiectasis; atelectasis (*a-* neg, *telos*, end, no expansion of ends). telangiectasis (sect. 23). (73), no expansion of ends).
emphysaein	inflate	emphysema.
eurys	wide	aneurysm.
meteorizein	to raise up	meteorism, abdominal distension, syn. tympanites
oidema	swelling	oedema.
varix, varicis, L.	dilated vein	varicose, varicocele.
coarctere, L.	to compress	coarctation of aorta.
phimosis	a muzzling	
stenosis	contraction	
stypticos	contracted	styptic.
systole	a placing together hence contraction (of heart walls).	

33. STIMULATION

agogos	leading	cholagogue, substance stimulating flow of bile (p. 29; sect. 9).
hormaein	to stir up	hormone.

34. CHANGE, MODIFICATION

meta-	change	metamorphosis; methaemoglobin, lit. changed haemoglobin; meta-

		stasis, lit. change in place; metaplasia, change from one kind of tissue into another.
para-	change	paratyphoid, lit. modified typhoid; paraesthesia, changed sensation.
amoiba	change	amoeba, amoeboid movements, here meaning change in shape.
tropos	turn	atropine (p. 22); sometimes used loosely for an ill-defined alteration, e.g. 'thyrotropic hormone of the pituitary'; ectropion, entropion, outward and inward turning of the edge of the eyelid.
divertere, L.	to diverge	diverticulum, lit. a small diversion.

35. GOODNESS, BADNESS; EASE, DIFFICULTY

eu-	well, good, hence easy, comfortable	eugenic, *genos* (sect. 22); euthanasia (*thanatos*, death); euthyroid.
dys-	difficulty	1. difficulty in performing a function; dysphagia, difficulty in swallowing (lit. eating); dysentery.
		2. pain in performing a function; dyspepsia, dysmenorrhoea.
malus, L.	bad	malformation; malabsorption.
cacos	bad	cachexia.

36. MOVEMENT, TRANSPORT

kinema	movement	kinaesthesia, sense of movement.
phora	movement	
phoreo	I carry, L. syn. *fero*	heterophoria, difference in movement of the two eyes; euphoria; epiphora, carry-

		ing over, i.e. overflow of tears; chromatophore; diaphoresis, carrying through, sweating.
rhoia **rheuma**	a flowing	rheumatism (p. 12); catarrh, flowing down; diarrhoea, flowing through; leucorrhoea; dysmenorrhoea; haemorrhoids; cholera, flowing of bile. (Note spelling -rrh- after prefixes.)
staxis	dripping	epistaxis.
diabetes	passing through, syphon	Word already used for the disease by later Greeks, perhaps because water passed through patients as though through a syphon
vagus, L.	wandering	the nerve is so called because of its wide distribution.
herpein	to creep	herpes.
serpere, L.		serpiginous (cf. serpent).
claudicare, L.	to limp	claudication.
dromas	a running	syndrome, a running together, concurrence of symptoms) (cf. hippodrome).
trechein	to run	trochanter, i.e. part used in running.
trochos	a wheel, pulley	trochlea.
decussare	cross like an X	decussate.
choreia	a dance	chorea, so-called from its epidemic form characterized by dancing movements.
pedesis	a leaping	diapedesis, passage of leucocytes through walls of capillaries.
osmos	thrust	osmosis.
clonos	violent movement	clonic contractions
rhexis **rhagia**	a bursting or bursting out	haemorrhage; karyorrhexis, bursting of nuclei. Menorrhagia, excessive loss

		during the menses: metrorrhagia (*metra*, uterus) loss independent of the menses.
deciduus, L.	falling off	decidua (cf. deciduous).
lapsus, L.	a fall	prolapse (cf. collapse).
procidere, L.	to fall	procidentia, syn. prolapse.
ptosis	a fall	symptom (lit. a falling together); visceroptosis, etc.
talipes	walking on the talus	
listhesis	a sliding	spondylolisthesis, sliding of one vertebra on the one below.
nictare, L.	to wink	nictitating membrane.
nystagmos	nodding	nystagmus, lateral movements of the eye.
kyma	wave	kymography.

37. SENSATION, FEELING

placebo, L.	please	lit. I will please; drug given to please the patient.
paregoreo	soothe (orig. exhort)	paregoric, a drug which soothes pain.
aesthesia	feeling	hyper-, an-, par- aesthesia, anaesthetics.
thymos		cyclothymia.
libido, L.	lust	
algos	pain	analgesia, neuralgia, proctalgia, etc.
angina, L.		from *angere*, strangle (cf. anger, anguish); also used of inflammation of throat in Ludwig's angina.
colicos		lit. relating to the colon, hence colic.
odyne		pleurodynia; acrodynia; anodyne, drug which relieves pain.
phobos	fear	photophobia; claustrophobia; agoraphobia (p. 13).

38. SPECIAL SENSES

phos, phot-	light	photography; photosensitive.
opsis	sight	optic; hemianopia, etc.
scopos	a view	microscope, etc.
acousis	hearing	acoustic; hyperacusis.
audire, L.	to hear	auditory (cf. audience).
olere, L.	to smell	olfactory.
osme	a smell	anosmia; parosmia.
geusis	taste	ageusia.
gustus, L.	taste	degustation; gustatory (lingual) nerve; (cf. disgust).
glycys	sweet	glucose; glycogen; glycosuria, etc.
oxys	bitter	oxygen, lit. acid-forming; oxyntic (sects 17 and 30).

39. CUTANEOUS SENSATIONS

excoriare, L.	to flay	excoriation, abrasion of skin as by scratching.
formica, L.	ant	formication, formalin, formaldehyde (formic acid originally obtained from ants).
prurire, L.	itch	prurigo, pruritus.
psora	itch	psoriasis.
scabere, L.	to scratch	scabies (but see p. 108)
tactus, L.	touched, from *tangere,* to touch	tactile.

40. MENTAL STATES

(See also sect. 37)

mens, mentis, L.	mind	mental, etc.
phren	mind	schizophrenia (sect. 26).
psyche	spirit, soul (p. 10)	
syncrasis	temperament (*crasis,* mixture)	idiosyncrasy; dyscrasia, lit. bad mixing (cf humours).
mnesis	memory	amnesia, loss of memory,

		anamnesia, history (lit. memory back or recollection: hence applied to medical history); mnemonic.
gnosia	knowing, recognizing	agnosia; astereognosis.
noiein	to think	paranoia.
phasis	speech	aphasia.
phone	voice	aphonia.
lalis	speech	dyslalia, echolalia.
graphe	writing	agraphia.
lexis	reading	alexia.
praxis	doing	apraxia.
lethargos	drowsy	lethargy.
narce	torpor	narcosis, narcotic.
hypnos	sleep	hypnosis, hypnotic.
caros		carotid (p. 16).
somnos, L.		somnolent.
coma	deep sleep	comatose.
sopor, L.		soporific.
moros	foolish	moron.

41. GROWTH, REPRODUCTION

physis	growth (also nature, whence many other words, p. 31).	apophysis, projection of bone not ossified separately; diaphysis, shaft of bone; epiphysis, separate ossification at the end; metaphysis, bone recently deposited on the diaphysial side of the epiphysial growth cartilage; hypophysis, lit. growth below, syn. pituitary.
blastos	germ, sprout	parent of mature cell, erythroblast; osteoblast; s p o n g i o b l a s t ; neuroblastoma.
germen, L.	bud	germinal, germ-cell, dysgerminoma.
oncos	growth	oncology, oncometer.

gone	seed	gonad; gonorrhoea.
semen, L.		seminiferous.
sperma, spermatos		spermatic; spermatozoa; azoospermia.
sporos		spore; sporadic, i e. scattered like seeds.
embryon	embryo	
anthos	blossom	exanthem, lit. a blossoming out, an infective disease with a rash.
cyesis	pregnancy	pseudocyesis, false pregnancy.
tocos	birth	oxytocin, lit. rapid birth, the pituitary secretion which stimulates the pregnant uterus to contract.
parere, L.	to bring forth	primipara, multipara, parturition.
gestare, L.	to bear	gestation.
gravidus, L.	heavy, i.e. pregnant	gravid uterus; primigravida.
pareunos	lying beside	dyspareunia (painful coitus).
genos	offspring	genetic, etc. (p. 84).
neos	new	neonatorum, of the newborn.
teras, teratos	monster	teratoma.

42. NUTRITION, DIGESTION, EXCRETION

trophe nourishment trophic ulcer, ulcer due to deficient nourishment. Usually used to signify the result of nourishment, i.e. growth, although the disturbance may not be caused by abnormal nourishment: atrophy, dystrophy, hypertrophy.

sitos parasite, something (or someone) getting food on the side at something (or someone) else's expense.

alimentum, L.	nourishment	alimentary.
pabulum, L.		
pepsis	digestion	peptic; dyspeptic; pepsin.
phagein	to eat	phagocyte, dysphagia, etc.
prandium, L.	mid-day meal	post-prandial.
ereptomai	I eat	erepsin.
macerere, L.	chew	macerate.
mandere, L.		mandible.
masesthai		masseter.
merycizein	chew the cud	merycism (habit of chewing regurgitated food).
trismus	gnashing	spasm of jaw muscles.
mylos	mill	mylo-hyoid.
mola, L.		molar.
orexis	appetite	anorexia.
opson	seasoning	opsonin.
dipsa	thirst	polydipsia, dipsomania.
expectorare, L.	to expectorate	lit. from the chest.
ptysis	a spitting	ptyalin, haemoptysis.
vomere, L.	vomit	
emeticos	provoking vomiting	emetic, haematemesis, hyperemesis.
chezo	defaecate	dyschezia.
enoureo	pass urine	enuresis.

43. CONSTRUCTION, DESTRUCTION, OBSTRUCTION

genea   race, family, offspring   This root has a very wide use in words meaning birth, family, cause, formation, origin, etc. e.g. hydrogen, oxygen, genetics. It is used both in active and passive: pathogenic, causing disease; iatrogenic, caused by doctors.

plasma   mould, matrix, *plassein,* to form   anaplasia, reversion to a more primitive tissue; aplastic, defective formation; hyperplasia, excessive formation; meta-

		plasia, change from one type of tissue to another; achondroplasia, no formation of cartilage; plastic surgery; neoplasm; protoplasm, etc.
synthesis	placing together	see thesis, sect. 23.
poiesis	a making	haemopoiesis.
bole	lit. a throwing, *ballein*, to throw	anabolism, building up; catabolism, breaking down; metabolism, exchange in building; embolus, something thrown in (also a name for the 'thrown in' extra day of leap year).
lysis	a breaking down, adj. lytic, *lyein*, to loose	analysis; catalysis; haemolysis; osteolytic. (A latinized form is *lues*, used rarely for syphilis, more commonly as the adj. luetic.)
clastos	broken, *clan*, to break	osteoclastic.
teirein	to break	lithotrite, instrument for breaking calculi.
infarctus, L.	stuffed up	infarct.
thrombos	plug	thrombosis.
detritus, L.	rubbed away	
obturare, L.	to stop up	obturator.

44. VIOLENCE, ATTACK

impetere, L.	to attack	impetigo.
lepsis	attack	epilepsy, etc.
agra	prey	podagra (*pous, pod-*, foot), i.e. gout; perhaps also pellagra (*pella*, skin).
pledge	blow	apoplexy (cf.E stroke); hemi-, di-; mono-, para-plegia.
angere, L.	to strangle	angina.
rabere	rave	rabies.

nocere, L.	to injure	innocuous; anoci-association; nociceptive (*capere*, L., to receive).
acerbus, L.	bitter	exacerbate.
trauma, traumatos	injury	traumatic.
colobos	mutilation	coloboma, defect of eye.
syncope	fainting	
toxicos	poisonous	orig. arrow-poison, from *toxon*, bow; toxic, toxaemia; antitoxin, etc. (cf. toxophily, archery).
virus, L.	poison	virulent.

45. PROTECTION

alexein	to protect	alexin (syn. complement).
antidon	given against	antidote.
ischein	to check	ischaemia, lit. checking of blood.
munitio, L.	a fortifying	immunity (L. *in*, not), fortifying against.
phylaxis	guard	prophylaxis, protection in advance; anaphylaxis (p. 30).

See also vaccination, inoculate (p. 15).

46. SOUNDS

aix, aigos	goat	aegophony.
amphoreus	jar	amphoric breathing.
crepitare, L.	rattle, creak	crepitation.
borborygmai	(onomatopoeic)	
fremitus	murmuring	palpable thrill.
gargarizein	(onomatopoeic)	gargle.
pectus, L.	chest ⎫	pectoriloquy.
loqui, L.	speak ⎭	
rhonchos	snore	rhonchus.
stertere, L.		stertorous.
tinnere, L.	ring	tinnitus.
tussis, L.	cough	pertussis, whooping cough.
tympanum, L.	drum	tympanum, eardrum; tympanites.

47. WASTING, DECAY, DEATH

cachexia	extreme wasting (*cacos*, bad; *hexis*, state).	
caries, L.	dry rot	
gangraina	gnawing	gangrene.
marasmos	wasting	marasmus.
phthisis	wasting	
tabes, L.	wasting	tabes mesenterica; tabes dorsalis, lit. wasting of the back; craniotabes, wasting of skull.
sepsis	putrefaction	septic; septicaemia.
sapros	putrid	saprophyte (plant living on decaying matter).
necros	dead	necrosis (a state of death); necropsy, seeing the dead.
ptoma	dead body	ptomaine.
sequestrum, L.	lit. something put aside	
thanatos	death	euthanasia.

48. PHARMACEUTICAL ABBREVIATIONS

aa., *ana*, of each (drug named).
a.c., *ante cibum*, before meals.
b.d., *bis die*, twice a day.
f., ft., *fiat*, let it be made.
garg., *gargarisma*, gargle.
guttae, drops.
haust., *haustus*, draught.
liq., *liquor*, solution.
lot., *lotio*, lotion.
mane, in the morning.
mist., *mistura*, mixture.
mitte (tales doses), deliver so many doses.
nocte, at night.
hac nocte, to-night.
p.c., *post cibum*, after meals.
p.r.n., *pro re nata*, when required.
q.s., *quantum sufficiat*, a sufficient quantity.
rep., *repetatur*, let it be repeated.

rep. ambo., repeat the two things.
rep. omnia., repeat everything.
sec. art., *secundum artem*, with pharmaceutical skill, *i.e.* giving the pharmacist a free hand.
s.o.s., *si opus sit*, if necessary (but see p. 99).
ss, *semis*, half.
syr., *syrupus*, syrup.
tab., *tabula*, tablet.
t.d.s., *ter die*, three times a day.
t.i.d., *ter in die*, three times a day.
troch., *trochiscus*, lozenge.
tr., **tinct.**, *tinctura*, tincture, solution in alcohol.

49. WORDS NOT TO BE CONFUSED

Aura, breeze or emanation, *aureus*, golden and *auris*, ear.
blast-, sprout, *clast-*, break and *plast-*, mould.
hebe, youth and *hebes*, dull.
hidros, sweat and *hydor*, *hydro-*, water.
homo, man and *homo*, *homeo*, same.
ileum, intestine and *ilium*, bone.
mens, mind and *menses*, menstrual flow.
mucus, *myxa*, mucus and *myces*, fungus.
os, *oris*, mouth and *os*, *ossis*, bone.
osteo-, bone and *ostium*, opening.
pes, *pedis*, foot and *pais*, *paidos*, child.
pyr-, from, *pirum*, pear and *pyr*, *pyros*, fire.
rickets and Rickettsia (a group of sub-bacterial organisms including those causing typhus named after the discoverer, H. T. Ricketts).
trop-, turn and *troph-*, nourishment.

PART IV

NON-CLASSICAL ORIGINS

The classical languages and their roots remain to this day the major source and model for the formation of medical words. But they are not the only source: the net spreads ever wider. There is a fair scattering of words from other European languages and a few Arabic, and an increasing number (especially for tropical diseases) nowadays from other languages of great diversity.

MODERN FRENCH

As indicated in an earlier section, it is often difficult with older words to know whether they arose directly from Latin or indirectly via French. The following list consists of more recent borrowings (mostly during the 1700s), and all retain the exact or nearly exact form of the original French. Only ergot, goitre, tissue and trocar have been so thoroughly accepted that their origin has been forgotten. Most of the rest retain some relics of the original pronunciation, and the italicized ones are clearly still regarded as foreign words.

Accoucheur; 'obstetrician'.

Ballotement; the bounce of a fetus away from a prodding finger: *balloter* is to play with a ball.

Bistoury; F. *bistouri*, 'scalpel': limitation of the name to the curved probe-pointed form is relatively recent.

Bougie; originally a wax candle (from the town Bougie in Algeria): still in France, and in England for a time, used in both senses.

Bruit; 'noise'.

Cancer *en cuirasse*; in both languages a cuirass was

close-fitting chest armour, originally of leather *(cuir)*: the skin infiltration in breast cancer obviously relates to the leather variety.

Chancre; L. *cancer:* used for both tumour and venereal sore in French, limited to the sore in English (see p. 104).

Contre-coup; brain damage opposite to the side of blow: in French in general use for rebound, backlash etc.

Curette; from F. *curer*, to clean out or dredge, hence a small spoon for scraping.

Débridement; in French means to unbridle, or medically to separate adhesions: the English usage for cleaning a wound probably derives from confusion with débris, which is a different word entirely (*briser*, to break; *brider*, to bridle).

Douche; 'shower' or 'spray'.

Ergot; 'cock's spur': the rye disease was so called from the appearance of the affected ears.

Fièvre boutonneuse; 'fever with a button': South African tick-bite fever, one of the scrub typhus group, the 'button' being a dark nodule at the site of the original bite.

Folie (*à deux* etc.); 'madness'.

Forme fruste; a disease incompletely manifested: the *fruste* means worn or defaced (like an old coin) rather than frustrated.

Goitre; rather surprisingly, a French word, from L. *guttar*, throat, through Provençal, for the enlarged thyroid gland. It is older than the others, first noted in English in 1625.

Grand mal, petit mal; used for the severe and mild forms of epilepsy, yet we never use '*mal*' alone for epilepsy – nor it seems, do the French.

Guillotine; Dr Guillotine, inventor of the prototype, has given his name to various instruments, especially one once much used for removing the tonsils.

Lavage; F. washing.

Legionnaire's disease; a severe form of pneumonia, due to a previously unrecognized form of bacillus (now called *Legionella*), which owes its name to an epidemic occurring in one hotel during a convention of American 'Legionnaires'. The newest name in this book. The English word is legionary.

Main en griffe; 'a claw hand', literally.

Massage; also means a shampoo and a rub-down for a horse in French.

Migraine; from Latin (He)micrania: adopted twice from French, in the middle ages as megrim, which was used for dizziness and whims and 'the vapours' so widely that the French form was re-introduced for the precise disease, with attacks of one-sided severe headache, visual disturbance and sickness. Megrim was a common enough term at least till the 1700s, and occurs occasionally as a medical term in the 1800s.

Râle (or rale); introduced by Laennec (of the stethoscope) for the more rattling of chest noises. The word in French, however, does not mean a rattle generally, only the death rattle or noises like it (or a corncrake).

Souffle; 'a breath, puff or blast': chiefly of the blowing noise heard over the pregnant uterus.

Tache (*cérébrale, noir* etc.); 'spot, stain or blemish': a common word in Middle English (Gawain's speech was 'teccheles', i.e. spotless) but lost, and re-introduced relatively recently in a few French expressions.

Tampon; ' plug': this also is a recent re-introduction, the original form tampion (or tompion) still being in use for a plug in the muzzle of a gun.

Tic and *tic douloureux;* respectively a twitch, and the painful disease trigeminal neuralgia: tic is said to be originally a bad habit of horses. The correct spelling of the neuralgia is *douloureux,* though the Latin is *dolor* and no other language introduces two u's. Strictly speaking, if the expression is used in English, and especially so long as more or less successful efforts are made to give it a French pronunciation, *doloureux* is a solecism.

Tissue: F. *tissu:* in the sense of woven material the word is old, but the medical sense for the main types of body constituent was newly imported after 1800.

Tourniquet; 'turnstile, roller, turnbuckle' etc., as well as our medical sense: from *tourner*, turn.

Trocar; F. *trocart*, originally *trois-carre*, 'three-sided': the sharp instrument used to introduce a cannula, originally three-sided and still often having a triangular point.

ITALIAN

Belladonna; *bella donna,* 'beautiful lady': the use for the nightshade is much older than for the drug obtained from it. Presumably the name derives from its use to enhance beauty by dilating the pupils, but there is some doubt about it.

Influenza; this is the ordinary Italian word for influence, extended originally to epidemics (astrological influence being assumed), then to one particular epidemic of influenza ('*the* epidemic') in 1743, and thereafter used for that disease. The French *grippe* ('grip, dislike') seems to be popular with several other languages, and has only recently died out·in English: the Spanish have the delightful *trancazo* ('hit with a truncheon').

Malaria; *mal' aria,* 'bad air': from the miasmas of the swamps thought to be the cause. The decline of Greece and Rome is often blamed on the spread of malaria, due either to ill-judged irrigation or the failure to maintain drainage.

Favism; *fava,* 'bean' (L. *faba*): the acute anaemia produced in carriers of glucose-6-phosphate dehydrogenase deficiency by eating beans, similar in nature to primaquine sensitivity. The skin disease favus is a quite different word, from the Latin for honeycomb.

Petechia; *petecchia,* 'spot': in English used only for flea-bite small haemorrhages in the skin. Note that -ia is the singular (pl. -ias): since the word is not Latin there is even less than usual justification for -iae – certainly none for -ia as plural with singular -ium!

Pellagra; *pelle agra,* 'rough skin' (probably): the disease caused by deficiency of the B vitamin nicotinamide, usually associated with poor maize diets, once common in the southern USA and Mediterranean countries.

Quarantine; *quaranta,* 'forty': from the forty days' quarantine once thought necessary for ships from plague areas.

SPANISH

It is noteworthy that nearly all these refer to tropical diseases, and are often derived originally from local languages. All of them are the normal names now used for these diseases in English.

Chiclero ulcer: leishmaniasis of the skin, from its prevalence in Mexican collectors of chewing gum or *chicle,* the latter being a Nahmatl word. (Rather grandly referred to as '*Enfermedad de los chicleros*' in one US textbook – *enfermedad* being infirmity.)

Dengue; the common, unpleasant, but rarely dangerous mosquito-borne fever of much of the tropics. The word means 'fastidiousness' in Spanish. Apparently an originally Swahili word 'dinga' was assimilated as 'dengue' by Spanish-speakers and 'dandy' by English-speakers in the West Indies (both senses were helped by the characteristic stiff neck), and the former has generally been adopted.

Erisipela de la Costa; 'Erysipelas of the coast': a form of onchocerciasis of Central America.

Espundia; muco-cutaneous leishmaniasis of tropical Latin America, (?) related to *espuma,* froth, scum.

Mosquito; 'little fly': Sp. *Mosca,* L. *musca,* fly.

Piedra; 'stone' (L. *petra*): a fungus infection producing stony hard nodules in the hair in tropical S. America and Indonesia.

Pinta; 'coloured spot' (L. *pincta,* painted): a non-venereal treponema infection of children from Mexico to the Amazon, produced scaly, bluish, skin lesions which leave white depigmented areas after healing: cf. US pinto for a piebald horse.

Quinine; from Sp. quina, from Quichuan *kina* or *kinkina,* bark.

Uta; Peruvian type of cutaneous leishmaniasis.

Verruga peruana; 'Peruvian wart' (Sp., not L. which would be *peruviana*): chronic bartonellosis; besides the nodular skin lesions there are visceral lesions producing long-lasting ill-health. Often referred to simply as verruga or verrugas.

GERMAN

In view of the dominant role in medical science played by Germans from about 1830 to 1930, it is surprising how few words we have adopted from them. Because they found it difficult to assimilate terms of Romance-classical origin into their language, they tended until recently to invent their own terms by agglutinating German words, and the results did not export easily. Oddly enough, though, they often wrote formal diagnoses and anatomical descriptions in strictly grammatical Latin. The international BNA system of anatomical nomenclature in its original form was typically and paradoxically German in its impossibly formal Latin.

Anlage; 'plan, foundation': the first recognizable signs of any structure in the embryo.

Ester; shortened from *essig-aether,* acid-ether; ethers being formed by 'condensation' of two alcohols and esters by similar union of acid and alcohol.

Gestalt; 'form': a term in psychology I confess to not being able to define.

Gitterzell; 'lattice-cell': the fat-laden scavenger cell seen in breaking-down brain tissue, so called from the lattice appearance seen when the fat droplets are dissolved out in making routine microscopic preparations.

Darmbrand; 'gut-fire': enteritis necroticans, severe local damage to small intestine caused by clostridia, very similar to Pigbel (p. 98).

Fleckmilz; 'speckled spleen': a rare form of necrosis of the spleen.

Kernicterus; 'kernel-jaundice': the yellow staining of nuclei ('kernels') in the brain in severely affected Rhesus babies. Notice the unassimilated (i.e. unaltered) state of the Latin inclusion *icterus*.

Magenstrasse; 'stomach street': the short route from entrance (cardia) to exit (pylorus) in the stomach, along the lesser curve.

Mast cell; 'over-fed cell': the German *Mastzell* is short for *gemästete Zell*, (the fatted calf was a *gemästete Kalb* or a *Mastkalb*), the name arising from the numerous granules with which the cell is stuffed.

ARABIC

The Arab empires of the middle ages, apart from occasional outbursts of fanaticism, cherished in their own translations much of the learning of the Greeks during a time when Europe suffered under relative barbarism and a church opposed to all learning not written in Latin. Arab contacts (with Spanish Jews prominent before the days of the Inquisition) played an important part in the revival of learning that led to the Renaissance. Once started, however, scholars preferred to go back to the original texts preserved by the Byzantine empire, and surprisingly little Arabic survives in medical use. Chemistry preserves a great deal more – e.g. sugar, alcohol, alkali, naphtha, natrium (sodium, Na) and kalium (potassium, K). Medical examples, old and new, are:

Basilic and cephalic veins; though these two words are obviously Greek, meaning 'of the king' and 'of the head' respectively, they are applied to two veins in the arms, and the names were given them by the Arabs on an erroneous view of their function.

Bejel; (modern): non-venereal and mild syphilis of children, in the middle east and neighbouring desert areas.

Elixir; *al-iksir:* originally the Arab version of the philosopher's stone.

Halzoun; (modern): infestation of the throat with liver-fluke larvas from eating infected raw liver: chiefly Syria.

Mater; dura and pia mater are obviously Latin, the 'hard and soft mothers' of the brain: it is, however, a literal translation of the Arabic, the use of 'mother' for a protective covering being a common arab idiom and reasonable enough, however unfamiliar.

Nuchal; *nukha,* 'spinal cord': nucha also meant spinal cord in English originally, though now used only for the nape of the neck.

Senna; *sana.*

Syrup; *sharab,* with variants and derivatives in most southern European languages: sherbet and the once-popular drink shrub come from the same source.

OTHERS

This miscellaneous collection shows how wide the net is now spread. Only a few are really familiar in this country, but none of them are trivial. All are used in English descriptions – which in practice in many cases means the only available proper descriptions – of the diseases concerned.

Ackee poisoning; Jamaican local name of the fruit.

Alastrim; (?)Brazilian: a mild form of smallpox.

Beriberi; Cingalese, *beri,* 'weakness', with intensifying re-duplication: thiamine (vit. B_1) deficiency in wet (cardiac), dry (neuritic) and cerebral (Wernicke's encephalopathy) forms: not rare in this country in alcoholics.

Betel nut; Malayalam (S. India) via Portuguese: a very wide-spread cause of mouth cancer in S. India and S.E. Asia among those who chew various mixtures containing it.

Buruli ulcer; (Uganda district name): skin ulcers due to a mycobacterium, best known of a group that includes swimming-bath ulcers.

Chutta cancer; the chutta (Hindi) is a coarse Indian cheroot smoked with the burning end in the mouth, and causing cancer of the palate.

Dhoti cancer; the *dhoti* (Hindi) is the long Indian loin cloth: with inadequate cleaning, skin cancer occasionally arises under it – chiefly around Bombay.

Jigger; West Indian local name, properly Chigoe, possibly from Spanish *chico*, small: a flea, the pregnant females of which penetrate the skin and produce local abscesses.

Itai-itai-byo; Japanese, 'painful disease': cadmium poisoning.

Kala-azar; Assamese, 'the black disease': visceral leishmaniasis, spread by sandflies, a severe general infection with massive spleen enlargement and a substantial death rate, commonest in India but widespread in the tropics. Why 'black' seems uncertain, unless it refers to its severity.

Kangri cancer; Hindi, from Kashmiri: the pot of burning charcoal worn under the clothes in cold uplands, occasionally producing local skin cancer.

Kuru; Papua New Guinea local name: a fatal brain infection with a slow virus, associated with cannibalism and now extinct.

Kwashiorkor; Ga tribe of Ghana, sense disputed, perhaps the weaning disease: severe malnutrition of young children with predominance of protein lack, seen most often after weaning (also *boufissure* (swelling) *d'Annam, culebrilla* (little snake?) and many other names).

Lassa fever; village name in Nigeria: a very severe virus infection caught from monkeys.

Loa loa; Congo local name: infection with a small worm that produces Calabar swellings in the skin and also involves the conjunctiva. Loa loa is a local reduplicated name: the worm is also called *Loa loa* in proper scientific fashion – genus *Loa*, species *loa* – and the disease is called loiasis.

Madura foot, Maduromycosis; district in Madras: a destructive infection of the foot. *Not* from Madura Island, off Java.

Mkar disease; district in Nigeria: a skin disease often mistaken for leprosy.

Mongolism; *Mongol* was Jenghis Khan's hordes' own name for themselves: trisomy 21, the commonest major chromosome disorder and the commonest single cause of mental defect. The facial resemblance between patients and real mongols is remote, and the term is the only survival of a desperate 1880-ish attempt to relate types of mental defect to the main human races.

Onyalai; East African local name: purpura affecting chiefly the mouth.

O-nyong-nyong; 'wrench-wrench', East African local name: one of at least forty different tropical diseases due to arboviruses: this one causes an epidemic fever with severe muscular pains.

Pibloktu; Eskimo name: Arctic hysteria, also a brain disease of dogs.

Pigbel; 'pork-belly', New Guinea Pidgin: enteritis necroticans, very common in the Papua New Guinea highlands, caused by feasting on large amounts of pork infected with Clostridia after long periods of low-protein diet.

Tanapox; Kenya: mild smallpox-like disease.

Tsutsugamushi fever; Japanese: mite-born scrub typhus.

Veld(t) sore; Afrikaans: cutaneous diphtheria, a relatively mild form of diphtheria common in many tropical areas. *Veld* is the current spelling in Dutch and Afrikaans: pronounced felt, however spelled.

ACRONYMS

We need look no further than the SPQR (*senatus populusque romanus*, senate and people of Rome) of the legions to realize that we did not invent acronyms, but they have certainly flourished greatly among us: the word itself ('tipname') is an invention of this century. In the strict sense of pronounceable words made out of initials – like Anzac (Australia and New Zealand Army Corps, one of the first really popular modern ones), radar, snafu, quango – they are not very common in medicine, but there are innumerable quasi-acronyms in the looser sense of sets of initials so well established that they are habitually used as words, often by people who have no idea what the initials stand for – DNA, RNA, ACTH, TSH, TID, BID, BBA, APH, HE, PAS, AFB,* (and see p. 87). SOS (give in emergency) is always interpreted in dictionaries as *si opus sit*, but I suspect that this is simply a Latin excuse for using the nautical distress signal (itself often construed 'save our souls') which like all international code signals of the kind is a purely arbitrary group of letters (dating from 1906 only) and not even a quasi-acronym in fact.

Here, however, are a few true medical acronyms; they have a strong microbiological bias:

Aflatoxin; Aspergillus FLavus toxin: of ground-nut poisoning.

---

* De-oxyribonucleic acid, ribonucleic acid, adrenocorticotrophic hormone, thyrotrophic hormone, *ter in die* (three times a day), brought in dead, born before arrival, antepartum haemorrhage, haematoxylin and eosin, paraminosalicylic acid and periodic-acid Schiff, acid-fast bacillus.

Apudoma; Amine Precursor Uptake and Decarboxylation -oma: tumour of APUD cells, which include argentaffine cells, islet cells, parafollicular cells, etc.

Arbovirus; ARthropod-BOrn virus: name, like several following, of a *group* of viruses: this one includes yellow fever, dengue, o'nyong-nyong and many others.

Bacon; Bleomycin, Adriamycin, CCNU, Oncovin, Nitrogen mustard – a drug combination used in cancer therapy. One of a number of such names for the numerous regimens (NB *regimens:* regimes is common but strictly wrong in this sense) being tried for this purpose, probably mostly ephemeral.

Dornase; De-Oxy-Ribo-Nucleic Acid lytic enzyme.

Echo-virus; Enteric Cytopathogenic Human Orphan: 'orphan' because when first discovered it was not known what diseases they caused (diarrhoea and meningitis, rarely serious).

Laser; Light Amplification Stimulated Emission Radiation.

Oncornavirus; *onco-* (tumour) RNA: leukaemia viruses of various animals.

Picornavirus; *pico-* (small) RNA: respiratory virus group including common cold.

Rad; Radiation Absorbed Dose	Measures of radiation dose used by radiotherapists.
Rem; Radiation Equivalent Man	
Rep; Radiation Equivalent Physical	

Reovirus; Respiratory and Enteric Orphan: (much as Echo).

Retrovirus; REverse-TRanscriptase-producing virus.

EPONYMS

The attachment of people's names to diseases and other things – *Bright's disease, Bell's palsy, Billroth operation, Koch's postulates, Coomb's test, Epstein-Barr virus, Conn's syndrome* – is a subject in itself. Though unfair in their distribution (no eponym celebrates Vesalius, or Paré, or Harvey, or Morgagni, or Virchow, or Fleming, or Kennaway) they do on the whole commemorate people and discoveries of importance, and an annotated dictionary of eponyms would be almost a history of medicine.

There are, however, too many of them, and no one can remember what they all mean. How many readers have any idea of the nature of the Klumpke, Kornzweig-Bassen or Melkerson syndromes? A normal name (e.g. inferior brachial plexus damage for the first, or even brachial plexus syndrome type II) would at least have been easier to recognize approximately for what it is. Eponyms are very low on the mnemonic grading in assessing usefulness of names. There is also the disadvantage that more than one eponym may be applied to one disease – e.g. *Graves* and *Basedow* (and at least two others) to hyperthyroidism, and *Brown-Kelly-Paterson* and *Plummer-Vinson* to iron deficiency anaemia with dysphagia.

Eponyms should be reserved as far as possible for conditions whose nature is so much in doubt that no exact name can safely be applied (*Hodgkin's disease* is a prime example) or where an adequately descriptive name would be far too long, as with some of the more complex and obscure syndromes, or the more recondite biochemical disorders: but in both these cases there perhaps need only be some drug-house-type verbal dexterity to solve the problem.

Eponyms of the simple forms exemplified by *Addison's disease* and *Burkitt tumour* (the 's is very much a matter of habit and preference) in which the name is used unaltered, are not the whole story. In many cases the name has been used as a root to make a new word. Examples are *pasteurization, addisonian* (of anaemia of true 'pernicious' type), *tyndalization* and *parkinsonism*. All these show the sign of full assimilation of an eponym into the language, loss of the capital letter. That this can happen without modification of the word is shown by *petri dish*, and by such non-medical words as wellington boot and tar macadam.

A few examples of this process are worth annotation: the first three have lost their capitals:

Galenical; a plant extract used as a medicine, from their formulation by Galen.

Masochism; from the Australian author Sacher-Masoch (died 1895), who described it: originally necessarily between the sexes.

Sadism; from the Comte de Sade, who practised and wrote about it. (Curious that both these two have literary origins rather than medical.)

Paracelsian; a follower of (or pertaining to) Paracelsus (d. 1541). Partly included as an excuse to note that despite a wide-spread opinion to the contrary, the word bombast has nothing to do with him, though his real name was probably Bombast von Hohenheim and the term would very well fit the inflated language with which he supported his revolutionary (but almost wholly erroneous) new system of medicine. It often has been ascribed to him and would, if true, be a kind of medical eponym. Bombast, however, means raw cotton wool used as a stuffing, and was used already both in literal and figurative senses in Elizabethan times – e.g. most appropriately of Falstaff.

We should finally not forget the Linnaean names of organisms which so often commemorate the microbiologists – sometimes two at a time, as in *Rickettsia prowazeki*, *Leishmania donovanii* and *Coxiella burnettii*.

PART V

MISCELLANY

This is a collection of notes by the present editor on various aspects of the English language and the ways it is used by doctors. I apologize for the dogmatic tone, but it makes for brevity; moreover, a clearly stated opinion, even if wrong, is often the quickest route to the truth, for it stimulates others to reasoned argument. One must believe something about the words one uses, and these are, at the very least, reasonable tenets till better truths appear.

The penultimate long section on US and UK English may seem out of place in a book on medical terms. Remember, however, that the people who benefit most from the existence of one language as an international means of communication (apart from such small groups as diplomats and airline pilots) are scientists, and of scientists, judged by the number of journals, medicals are responsible for by far the largest amount of such communication. Given then the convenience of having one's native tongue as the international language, it follows that English-speaking doctors have, of all people, a special interest in maintaining the unity and effectiveness of English.

Some of the notes are based in part on contributions to the *Lancet*'s Medical Idioticon column of the early 70s.

DICTIONARIES

Dictionaries have an almost divine authority in too many people's minds: they think that not only is what they say necessarily true, but it must be accepted as up to date even fifty years after it has been printed. Dictionaries are written by men, who may make errors and may have prejudices, and it is altogether impossible for even the largest and best-edited of them to include every possible word of every trade and every fashion in speech, or to be more up to date than some substantial number of years before the actual time of printing. Nearly all dictionaries, however, pander to our love of certainty; nearly always their implied message has been "This is the right way to use this word: anyone who uses it otherwise is an uneducated peasant or, worse, a foreigner." Johnson and Webster are great and successful examples of this didactic approach. But it is no accident that the dictionary with most real authority now in any language, the O.E.D., disclaims all authority for itself or its editors, simply recording how and when words have been used in practice in written English since English began. Only after browsing in its pages can one realize how much words change in sense over the centuries, how often the same word is used in different senses by different professions, often unknown to each other (umbilicus has mathematical and botanic senses quite different from ours, and neoplastic can mean 'according to the school of Mondriaan'); how nearly hopeless, too, it is to question any usage, however strange or illogical it may seem, once it has been accepted by any large body of speakers.

CARCINOMA, CANCER, CHANCRE, CANKER, CARCINOMA-IN-SITU

Here is a wonderful example of the independence of meaning from etymology. All the first four are etymologically the same word, yet who would pass a medical student now who confused them? *Carcinoma* is the Greek for crab, and they applied the name to the few superficial malignant tumours (breast and skin almost exclusively) that they could recognize. Rome used its own word *cancer* for both senses. Thence came the French word *chancre* and the English *canker* for any chronic ulcer, including malignancies. About 1600, when superficial malignancies were beginning to be more surely separated from other ulcers, cancer was adopted from the Latin in that specific sense (perhaps via its adoption a little earlier for the zodiac sign) and its use thereafter simply reflected growing understanding of that disorder. Carcinoma was at first little more than a euphemism for cancer, and it is only in the last thirty years that the more specific use has been widely accepted, limiting it to malignant epithelial tumours. Chancre and canker remained non-specific at first, but the French word, perhaps from anti-gallicism ('the French disease'), became limited to a venereal sore (though in French it continued to be more widely used, and only recently ceased to be used for cancer). Canker is now (if it is a medical term at all) limited to cancrum oris, though it still serves for various veterinary and horticultural diseases. The poor crab has now all but lost its hold on the word, though it still has claims on the zodiac sign, and the French words *cancre* and *carcin* refer to kinds of crab.

On quite another tack (an odd expression, by the way, since there are only two possible tacks, port and starboard), the term *carcinoma-in-situ* is worth considering. It has performed a most valuable function in frightening conservative gynaecologists into treating cases of pre-cancer of the uterine cervix adequately. Yet it is a misnomer: the lesion is not even a tumour, and by definition it is not invasive; there is no possible definition of carcinoma of any use to histopathologist and clinician that does not include invasiveness. It is, of course, simply the latest stage of *premalignant* (i.e. preinvasive) epithelial change. Again use is more valid than argument: the word is useful and may stand. But do not dissect it into its parts and say the lesion must *because of its name* be a tumour and malignant. And be very wary of indiscriminate use outside the cervix.

HOMOEOPATHY

Nowadays the ending -pathy (encephalopathy, nephropathy, mastopathy), nearly always means 'disease of', a convenient expression that does not commit one to any particular kind of disease. From this point of view homoeopathy should mean 'disease of the same thing', which is absurd. But just as in the early 1800s, when Hahnemann introduced the idea, there were so few genuinely useful drugs known (Jesuit's bark, opium, lime juice, digitalis – and what else?) that his new hypothesis was at that time well worth a trial, so also the word at that time had different connotations. It meant something very much the same as sympathy, a similarity of feeling: he treated disease with minute doses of drugs that in normal doses caused effects similar to those of the disease.

The Greek *pathos* had two related senses, of suffering and of feeling. In the first sense it came to be used of disease, Galen using *pathologikos* for the science of disease and *pathognomonikos* for a skilled diagnostician, and this is the usual medical sense of the root now. But until recently the ending -pathy (sympathy, telepathy, empathy) referred to the 'feeling' sense only.

The word homoeopathy had something of a vogue (Oliver Twist received food in homoeopathic doses in 1838) and was sufficiently misunderstood for it to be supposed that the -pathy referred to treatment. Every popular new treatment was so labelled – hydropathy (there were still fashionable hotels called Hydropaths when I was young), balneopathy, osteopathy, photopathy, etc. It is all the more remarkable that this sense has been all but forgotten (-therapy has taken its place, and who now knows why an osteopath is so called?) and the less confusing 'disease of' sense replaced it within a generation. There is no evidence that etymological considerations played any part in this.

The short list above of effective medicines available in Hahnemann's day suggests one curious thought. To that list there had just been added a totally new kind of agent – Jenner's vaccine. If anything fits the definition of a homoeopathic remedy, it is surely a live vaccine – it works in the minutest of doses, and its effects mimic those of the disease. And Jenner's vaccine can claim to be the most powerful medicine yet invented – the only one that has totally eradicated a major disease. If only Hahnemann had concentrated on that!

HYPER AND HYPO

I have put up this argument before, and no one listens, but perhaps it's worth another airing. These two excellent prefixes have one major defect; they sound almost alike in most people's mouths (a good rolled Scots r helps). They need not be. Until some time last century, hypo- was pronounced hippo- in English. The O.E.D. (the relevant part appeared in 1899) gives hippo- for preference, but admits the south of England was then switching. Hypocrite is now the only survivor of the original version. Is this not a sad degeneration of a useful distinction? When I remember, I say hippoglycaemia, but no one copies me, alas!

MOLES AND NAEVUSES

It is rather sad that the word mole is dropping out of medical use – chiefly, I suppose, from the love of learned-looking words with diphthongs in them but also because of mole (2) and mole (3). Our mole (1) is much the oldest, very Old High German in origin, meaning originally a spot of any kind (iron-mould is the same word, falsely assimilated to mould). Mole (2) for the animal, the mouldiwarp, is Dutch and mole (3), the breakwater, is Latin. There was once a 'French mole' which sounds as though it was a sebaceous cyst of the scalp lifting up the scalp, hair and all, like a mole-hill – an interesting concurrence of two of the senses. (Where hydatidiform mole fits all this I do not know – certainly it corresponds to none of the three senses already given. Oddly enough, none of the O.E.D.'s references under hydatidiform include the word mole – only disease or tumour of the chorion, all from the 1800s.)

Naevus is plain Latin, with no Greek precursor. (Modern Greek has *kreatoelia*, a 'flesh olive' and also *theloma*, a 'nipple-like' tumour.) It was first noted in 1693, and so is very much a newcomer. Since the word is used of two wholly distinct lesions, the vascular and the pigmented naevuses (or moles), it is rather a pity that the two words could not be divided between them. But naevus seems to have pre-empted both. Though it was not until last century that they were properly separated (curiously enough, for they are not usually hard to distinguish even when they are small), accurate early descriptions of naevuses seem usually to be dealing with the vascular form; while the use of 'naevus-cell' for the characteristic melanocytes of the pigmented form is very well established.

It will be a sad day when Viola's 'My father had a mole upon his brow' needs a commentator to explain he was not wearing a mouldiwarp or a breakwater. A small melanocytic mole one supposes – but did it go malignant? "My father had a mole upon his brow. And died...." that is the way Viola continues. Though, of course, malignant melanomas of the face are rare until old age, and as he died on Viola's thirteenth birthday he was unlikely to be very old.

SCABS AND SCABIES

Talking of Shakespeare ... it is midnight in Messina: the watch are wooing sleep on the church bench. Enter severally the two assistant villains. Borachio, the leading spirit but also the drunker of the two, calls Conrade twice.

Conrade. Here man, I am at thy elbow.
Borachio. Mass and my elbow itched, I thought there would a scab follow.

It seems unlikely, with millions of words written about Shakespeare every year, that this has not been noticed before, but, surely, is not Borachio referring to scabies? An itching followed by a scab, and exactly in the right place; what else could it be? Coriolanus also, in his first speech, seems to be thinking less precisely along the same lines:

> ... you dissentient rogues,
> That, rubbing the poor itch of your opinion,
> Make yourselves scabs.

Scab and scabies are totally distinct in origin, scab being Scandinavian (modern Swedish *skabb*), for skin disease, especially with pustules or itch. Scabies is Latin also for skin disease (*scabere* to scratch: cf. scabrous). The two terms were soon mixed up, and the word itch involved also, so that (while many skin diseases must have been confused together) it is likely that in Elizabethan times what we now call scabies was common and that anything described as the scab or the itch was as likely as not to be scabies; one would expect the word scabies to be used only by professionals, though not necessarily much more exactly. (Shakespeare does not use it, and elsewhere he uses itch only for the sensation and scab only as a term of more or less jocular abuse.) Borachio's jest is surely a typical Shakespearian triple play on the word scab as the disease, as the lesion expected on his elbow and as a highly appropriate appraisal of the third-rate knave Conrade by his wide-boy senior. It is also an example of the exact observation with which our bard basted on his fragments of medical knowledge.

ORTHOPOD

This slang expression for an orthopaedic surgeon is a rare example of an etymological conscience actually affecting the language. Orthopaedics is a strange word, meaning literally the straightening of children (G. *orthos*, straight, *pais, paidos,* a child): it was first used in English apparently in the title of the Royal Orthopaedic Hospital in 1835, where they dealt at first chiefly with club foot. The speciality rapidly widened, but kept the name, though now it is very inappropriate. The Greek *paid-* root appears in its Latin form as paedagogus, which became pedagogue in English (Caxton in 1483). The diphthong (seen also in paediatrics) is the result of copying the usual process whereby the Greek ai- became Latin ae- (as in aetiology and anaesthetic): it is perhaps a pity that Caxton's example was not followed.

The -pod in orthopod, of course, means foot – G. *poys,*

podos – as in podagra (gout), decapod (lobster) and podiatrics, which is I gather the new name for up-market chiropodists. But there is, in fact, an old Greek word, *orthopodeo,* to walk straight or upright, which makes an orthopod an upright walker – at least as proud a label as orthopaedic.

SCAN

Our hospital physicists seem to have adopted this word for pretty well any kind of examination of a patient with one of their instruments. A Gamma-camera, for instance, sits stock still absorbing γ-rays through the holes in its massive lead lens (even less like a lentil than a glass lens), and 'scans' the object no more than an ordinary photographer's camera, yet the physicist calls it a scan. Originally, of course, there *was* a scan: there was a single detector and it moved in a regular pattern over the area concerned, building up a picture of the isotope distribution in the tissues from the rays emitted, and that kind of regular patterned movement was reasonably described as scanning. The name has stuck when the movement has gone.

The word has a strange origin, from the Latin *scandere,* to climb (as in ascend). The Romans appear to have beaten time with their feet when listening to poetry, like unsophisticated music-lovers today. Hence the word 'foot' for the stress-divisions of a line of verse, and hence also, because the foot-stamping suggested climbing, of the use of *scandere* for the process of checking that this line had the right number and kind of feet (scansion). That came into English as scan – one scans a line of verse to see if it scans – and only after this did scan come to be extended to careful visual inspection. It retained perhaps a faint sense of running along a horizontal line: 'scanning the horizon' has a distinct if distant resemblance to running the eye along a line of print. So when a word was needed for the systemic geometrical pattern used in searches by radar equipment, scan seems to have been adopted at once as the obvious word. It is equally used now for various other instruments, including the line by line technique of the TV screen, and seems to be much more popular than the word raster (L. for rake) which was invented to describe the systemic coverage of the surface of the cathode ray tube by the electron beam. All those schoolboys, Roman and British, who were bullied into learning scansion would surely wonder to see how far the word has travelled: but they would, I think unhesitating, rate the use for a γ-camera, or any other stationary device, as in the class of doggerel!

JAUNDICE

This is an old borrowing from French (*jaune,* yellow, *jaunisse,* yellowness: the d in English is an intrusion), unusual among such borrowings in having no classical antecedants (G. *ikteros,* L. *icterus:* and yellow is G. *kitrinos* and L. *flavus*). There was a time when in addition to the yellow, black and green varieties (which one still hears of) there were also a white jaundice (chlorosis) and a blue jaundice (cyanosis). Since chlorosis is the green sickness of iron deficiency anaemia, to call it white jaundice is a singular confusion of colours – an example of the dangers of neglecting etymology too rashly. A jaundice can be yellow or greenish, but surely nothing else.

There is a tale that *ikteros,* the original Greek word, was before that the name of a yellow bird. If you had jaundice, you only had to see an *ikteros* to be cured: the bird it was that died.

THE GUT

It is an interesting exercise to travel down the gut, observing the variety of sources from which we get our names.

Oesophagus is good ancient Greek, though no one knows why the Greeks called it that. *Oisophagos* should mean something that eats *Oisos,* and what *oisos* is remains a mystery.

Cardia is simply the Greek for heart. It was used for the hither end of the stomach by Hippocrates himself. It suggests a belief that the connexion was more than mere propinquity. Is there a hint in the word cordial (L. *cor, cordis*) for a 'heart' medicine? (Beatrice was recommended to "get you some of this distilled Carduus Benedictus, and lay it to your heart".) Since cordials are carminatives that presumably relieve some dyspepsias referred to the heart area, may it have been that the speed of their action suggested to Hippocrates that they acted through the cardia?

Stomach looks like an honest old English word in a string of classical imports, especially as gastric looks like Latin. In fact stomach is classical, derived from *stoma*, mouth and originally referred to the throat, but moved downwards with time, becoming as *stomachus* the ordinary Latin for stomach. Gastric is Greek with no Latin intermediate, and ventral Latin with no Greek original: both meant belly and its contents generally, and were then as likely to be used of the uterus as the stomach. Venter, in fact, long survived in the uterine sense in the curious legal usage 'a son by a second venter' – i.e. by the second of two fertile wives.

Duodenum; the twelve-inch organ. L. *duodecim*, twelve, *duodeni* twelve at a time: invented about 1400.

Jejunum; L. *ieiunus*, fasting or empty – as in jejune, 'empty-headed'. As explained in 1541: "because it is always empty for the great multitude of mesenteric veins that be about it continually sucking it".

Ileum; L. *ile*, pl. *ilia*, guts, loins; the present form results partly from confusion with G. *eileos*, colic, whence ileus. The relation to *ileum*, which also meant flank at first, before its present sense for the bone, is not clear.

Caecum; L. the blind thing. In man it is no more a blind end than the fundus of the stomach, and the name presumably derives from the much more prominent structure seen in herbivores.

Colon; G. *kolon*, food, guts, large intestine. No Latin form. The punctuation mark comes from a different Greek word, *kōlon* (with omega instead of omicron for the first o) which meant limb and hence part of a sentence and has nothing to do with the gut. But oddly enough modern Greek uses the word only for the large intestine and spells it with an omega: maybe it is a re-introduction from English. (The French *colon* for an Algerian colonist is apparently not an obliquely scatological insult: it is old French and older Latin *(colonus)* for a farmer/settler).

Rectum; Latin, the straight thing (not very, but more so than the sigmoid, the S-shaped thing). Formerly the fundament and the longanon, both Latin also.

So, not one good Anglo-Saxon word among them. *Intestines* is mere Latin too, the 'insides'. Even *bowels* is Latin, from the same sausage source as botulism. '*Gut*' is good old English, however, usually in the plural guts. O.E.D. says "formerly, but not now, in dignified use with regard to man". Presumably the existence of a very dignified journal called simply '*Gut*' (surely the shortest journal title anywhere ever) will change that judgement.

ENGLISH AND AMERICAN

Some may wonder why in Part IV there are no words derived from our major ex-colonies – US, Canada, Australia and New Zealand and anglophone South Africa. The answer is simple. What they speak are not only not *foreign* languages, they are not in any important sense separate languages at all. This is obvious enough to a Frenchman, say, but for the British and the Americans in particular, it needs re-stating.

Which of the two speaks real English? Neither, or if you prefer, both. England claims the original invention and the name, US claims the more active recent development and the larger number of current speakers. Neither argument is worth much. Arguments as to where the 'best' English is spoken are pointless – Oxford, Inverness, Philadelphia, Harvard, Melbourne, the BBC news studios: the average foreigner could barely tell them apart. To all such arguments I put in a counter claim for the Tyneside dialect. English is after all the language of the Angles, not the Saxons or the Jutes, and that rules out all southern English dialects: the baleful influence of the Saxons is shown in all Angle areas south of Durham by the dropping of h's: the northernmost Angles are now lowland Scots. So the true Anglian English is spoken now only in the small enclave of the northeast of England. Q.E.D! (You will have inferred by now that I am by birth a Geordie.) An absurd argument, of course, but no more absurd than any of the other arguments as to who talks 'real' English or the 'best' English.

A language is one language if it has a common form in which all literate speakers are immediately intelligible to each other, both in speech and print. This allows for the existence of many *dialects* which may not be mutually intelligible. I have observed a Canadian visitor in doubt as to whether a Glasgow bus conductor might not be talking Gaelic, and a group of Stamford students to whom I had been talking with ease became suddenly unintelligible when they dropped into campus argot in talking to each other. But the written English of medical journals printed anywhere in the world hardly varies, and even in speech a sentence or two to adjust the ear to the speaker's mannerisms is all one needs for nearly all English-speaking medicals. With areas such as India where a large number of people speak it among themselves as a common language but it is now the mother tongue of few, the adjustment needed is greater, but still not much: the average Indian doctor coming here speaks a version far less deviant than our hospital porters among themselves.

There are, of course, extreme deviant forms of English like the various pidgin and creole forms. New Guinea pidgin for instance consists mostly of recognizable English words but uses Melanesian sentence structure and concepts: it needs to be learned as a foreign language – relatively easily, but still learnt. That, however, is another story. The English of the main body of educated English speakers in general, and of medical workers when talking about medicine in particular, is one language.

The practical effect of this is that it is not only useless, but also improper, for anyone in this country to reject words or idioms simply because they are American – and vice versa. 'Americanism' is a reasonable description of a term originating in or for the time being more common in the US: it is not a term of abuse. The same applies to 'Briticism'. If a scientific term, wheresoever invented, proves useful to English speakers, it will become English. If a useful or vivid expression from local dialect or professional jargon is picked up by educated speakers anywhere, it will spread without reference to national boundaries. Like people, a word is good or bad according to the way it behaves in practice, and the land of its birth is irrelevant.

WEBSTERISMS. Noah Webster (1758–1843) of Webster's Dictionary (or Dictionaries – he seems to have a divided estate these days) was the best lexicographer of English between Samuel Johnson and Sir James Murray, but did the language one major disservice. His career was founded on a successful spelling book, and he was a rabidly jingoist American patriot. Deciding that American ought to be recognizably different from English, he contrived a set of spelling reforms – color for colour, center for centre, ax for axe, defense for defence, woolen for wollen, skillful for skilful, check for cheque, etc. – and browbeat his countrymen into accepting them. The process pretty well stopped there, fortunately, and to this day the only way you can recognize with certainty that you are reading an article from the *New Eng. J. Med.* and not the *Lancet* is the thin scatter of Webster-style spellings.

There is nothing intrinsically wrong with the changes. The trouble is that they are so trivial, a mere petty minuscule tinkering with the great spelling problem, that they make no real difference to the labour of learning to spell, and have no other use. They stand as a memorial to the brief period of misunderstanding during which America lost the British Empire, forming a permanent nuisance without any countervailing advantage. It is a pity that they should be a great man's most conspicuous memorial. Why could he not have tried for something really useful, like straightening out all our crooked irregular verbs?

DIPHTHONGS. This argument is particularly relevant to medicine in the matter of the many medical terms that contain diphthongs in the original and in most languages but have lost them in the US. Curiously enough, there is more justification for some of these than most anglophiles realize.

What seems to have happened is that when Greek words were adopted into Latin their diphthongs often became single vowels. The words were first found in English in the Latin form, but at the Renaissance the Greek originals were recognized, and the diphthongs were mostly restored. The effect was so picturesque and learned-looking* that some quite unjustified forms appeared. The following list is all those I know of, though there may well be more.

(a) **Fetus,** *not* foetus: this is a straight Latin word, as the f shows. There is no Greek precursor.

(b) **Hydrocele,** *not* hydrocoele: from the Greek word *kele* a tumour or hernia, the ending having been later extended to mucocele, etc. No relation to coelom.

(c) **Leucopenia,** *not* leucopoenia: from Greek *penes*, to be poor, not Latin *poena*, penalty – and so, of course, in other -penia words.

(On leuco- or leuko- the argument is evenly balanced: the Greek is *leukos*, white, but the third letter of the Greek alphabet, gamma, always becomes g (gonad, twice in gynaecology), and kappa in consequence can become either

---

* The printing of diphthongs with a ligature (as in anæmia) is a quaint survival still dear to the *Lancet,* which has done enough pioneering to be allowed one antiquarian foible.

c or k, but most often c in Romance languages. The US leukocyte probably owes more to the influx of German pathologists than to Webster.)

The trouble about using this etymological argument to support Webster-style spellings is that etymology favours far more diphthongs than it rejects. Oedema, haemorrhage, aetiology, poietic, caecum, anaesthesia, amoebic, diarrhoea, gynaecology, homoeostasis, morbus caeruleus, for instance, all have impeccable classical antecedents. Oesophagus has an odd twist: there is no doubt of the classical form (oi-), but the mediaeval form *ysophagus* represents apparently one mediaeval way of coping with Greek oi- and *could* be held to justify esophagus.

The US spelling is therefore 'correct' in a few cases, the British in most. But, as this book has been at pains to demonstrate, etymology has little authority against established usage. Both spellings are correct in their own country, unfortunately.

Oddly enough, we need go no further than Phoenix, Arizona, to see that not all American diphthongs are reformed. A short search in Merriam-Webster found no exception to the rule that proper names follow the English rule (rather than the American or the original language) – e.g. Aesculapius, Aesop, Oedipus, Phoebus. This applies even when the names are absorbed into other words – aesculapian, oedipal, phoenician, daedalian. And in spite of pediatrics, one finds paedomorphic. Alas for consistency!

I hope the ultimate solution will not be simple submission to US numerical superiority. We ought to find a way of splitting the difference. Webster worked in part by bullying the printer-publishers of his day: could not perhaps the great publishing houses agree on a mid-Atlantic standard?

There is no solution in the way of true phonetic spelling. There could not possibly be an internationally agreed single form that covered all national variations in pronunciation: the language would simply fall apart into its dialects. We are stuck with written English basically as it stands, and have to make the best of it. Remember that the only language which is spoken by more people than ours – Chinese – shares with us two other distinctive features – an even simpler grammar, and an even greater divorce of written and spoken forms.

A FEW PRIVATE BÊTE-NOIRS

(a) People who argue about the plural of words like bête-noir (see p. 43).

(b) People who use the word parameter when they mean a variable, or when they mean almost nothing at all ('the parameters are favourable').

(c) People who pronounce polycythaemia as though it had a -th- sound in the middle, when it is clearly cyt-haem.

(d) People who argue *ad nauseam* about the niceties of language. It is a tool, not a decoration: if it gets across what you mean to the people it's meant for, it's good enough. Only things that destroy its efficiency wantonly, and especially that affect its international currency, are worth worrying about: and even there by the time the change is noticeable it is usually too late to do anything about it. Only one thing is certain about a living language: it will stay alive only as long as it retains the ability to change – and to change far further and far faster than any right-minded citizen could possibly accept as reasonable.

INDEX

Especially for references in Part III, where multiple, closely related words occur at one point in alphabetical order (such as *pepsis* and pepsin, or autologous and autogenous), not all the words are given in the index. It is often, therefore, worth looking up similar words if the one wanted is not in the index.

The lists of prefixes and suffixes on pages 27–29 have not been indexed.

Foreign words, or words generally treated as foreign, are shown in italics. But when English and foreign words of identical spelling occur in the text, they have been indexed under the same heading, and not in italics.

A-, 61
aa, 87
abbreviations, x, 87
abdomen, 20
abscess, 20
a.c., 87
acanthos, 68
acapnia, 56
accoucheur, 89
acerbus, 86
acetabulum, 60
achalasia, 77
achlorhydria, 61
achylia, 57
acinus, 73
ackee, 96
acne, 20, 68
acousis, 81
acromegaly, 71
acromion, 71
acron, 71
acronyms, 99–100
ACTH, 99
actinomycosis, 35, 60
acutus, 76
adamantinoma, 67
Adam's apple, 22
addisonian, 101
Addison's disease, 101
aden, 45

adenoid, 49
adeps, 60
aditus, 54
adnexa, 74
adventitius, 70
aegophony, 86
-aemia, 8, 9
aer, 55
aerophagy, 56
aesculapian, 117
aesthesia, 80
aetiology, 32
AFB, 99
afferent, 27
aflatoxin, 99
agammaglobulinaemia, 56
age, 70–1
agglutinate, 27
agglutination, 60
agnogenic, 34
agnosia, 82
-ago, 34
agoges, 77
agoraphobia, 13
agra, 85
air, 56
aither, 56
aix, 86
ala, 48

alastrim, 96
albumen, 36, 60
albuginea, 60
albus, 66
alcohol, 95
alexin, 86
algos, 80
alimentum, 34
alkali, 95
allantois, 48
allelomorph, 70
allergy, 40, 70
allos, 70
alopecia, 16, 68
alopex, 68
alveolus, 52
amauros, 66
amblyopia, 67
ambo, 62
amenorrhoea, 75
American, 113–18
Americanisms, 115
amnesia, 82
amnion, 20
amoeba, 78
amphoric, 86
amphoreus, 52, 86
ampi, 62
ampulla, 52
amylase, 60

119

INDEX

an-, 61
anaemia, 9, 61
anaesthetics, 80
analgesia, 80
analysis, 30, 85
anamnesia, 82
anaphylaxis, 30, 86
anaplasia, 84
anastomosis, 55
ancone, 45
aneurysm, 64, 77
angeion, 51
angina, 80, 85
angioma, 51
Angles, 114
Anglo-Saxon, 2, 3
animals, 58–9
Animal Spirit, 11
aniso-, 63
ankylosis, 64
anlage, 94
anodyne, 80
anomaly, 70
anopheles, 15
anorexia, 84
anosmia, 81
ansa, 48
anthos, 83
anthrax, 16, 60
anthropos, 70
antibodies, 42
antidote, 86
antipyretic, 75
antron, 52
anus, 47, 64
aorta, 20
APH, 99
aphakia, 60
aphasia, 82
aphonia, 82
aphrodisiac, 22
aphtha, 69
apnoea, 11, 56
aponeurosis, 13
apophysis, 82
apoplexy, 85
apothecary, 31
approximation, 74
apudoma, 100
aqua, 58
Arabic, 95–6
arachne, 55

arachnoid, 18, 49, 55
arbor, 73
arboviruses, 98, 100
Arctic hysteria, 98
areola, 13, 50
argentaffine, 100
argentum, 66
argyros, 66
Aristotle, 10
arrangement, 73–4
arthritis, 34
arthron, 45
articulatio, 45
arytaenoid, 49
ascaris, 48
ascos, 52
-asis, 35
aspergillus, 99
asphyxia, 18, 76
assimilation, 26
astereognosis, 82
asthenia, 77
asthma, 56
astigmatism, 72
astragalus, 20
astrocyte, 65
atavism, 70
ataxia, 72
atelectasis, 77
ater, 66
atheroma, 18
athetotic, 72
atlas, 22
atmos, 56
atrabilious, 12, 66
atresia, 55
atrium, 13, 52, 66
atrophy, 83
atropine, 22, 78
attack, 18, 85–6
audire, 81
aura, 56, 87
aureus, 66, 88
auricle, 13, 50
auris, 47, 88
autism, 69
autonomic, 69
autos, 9
axon, 48
azotaemia, 56
azoospermia, 83
azygos, 63

BACILLUS, 50
bacon, 100
Bacon, Francis, Lord
  Verulam, 6
bacterium, 51
badness, 78
balanos, 45
ballotement, 89
balneopathy, 106
bartonellosis, 94
barus, 67
Basedow's disease, 101
basilic, 96
BBA, 99
b.d., 87
bejel, 96
belladonna, 92
Bell's palsy, 100
beriberi, 96–7
betel nut, 97
bête-noirs, 118
bi-, 62
Bibles:
  Coverdale's, 5
  Luther's, 5
  Wyclif's, 4
biceps, 46
BID, 99
bigeminal, 63
bile:
  black, 12
  yellow, 11–12
bilis, 56
Billroth operation, 100
bistoury, 89
blast-, 88
blastos, 82
blennorrhoea, 57
blennos, 57
blepharon, 45
blood, 11
bole, 85
bombast, 102
Boorde, Andrew, 6
borborygmos, 86
bothrios, 52
bothyros, 73
botulism, 113
boufissure, 97–8
bougie, 89
bous, 58
bowels, 113

brachys, 64
bradycardia, 76
bradys, 76
breakwater, 107
breath, 56
Breviarie of Health, 6
brevis, 64
Bright's disease, 100
Briticism, 115
bronchiectasis, 77
bronchiole, 50
Brown-Kelly-
    Paterson's
    disease, 101
bruit, 89
bubo, 68
bucca, 47
buccinator, 15
bulla, 68
buphthalmos, 58
Burkitt tumour, 101
bursa, 52
Buruli ulcer, 97
byssos, 60

CACOS, 78
cachexia, 78, 87
caecum, 15, 112
caecus, 71
caesarian section, 22
calabar swellings, 98
calcaneus, 48
calcar, 48
calcarine, 48
calcification, 60
calculus, 50
callus, 67
calor, 75
calx, 60
calyx, 52
cancellus, 55
cancer, 58, 104
cancre, 105
cancrum oris, 105
canis, 58
canker, 104, 105
capillary, 69
capillus, 69
capitellum, 50
capnos, 56
capsule, 51
caput, 46

caput medusae, 22
carbuncle, 16, 60
carcin, 105
carcinogenic, 39
carcinoma, 58, 104, 105
carcinoma-in-situ, 104, 105
carcinos, 69
cardia, 11/12, 46, 95
caries, 57
carina, 48
caro, 46
caros, 82
carotid, 16
cartilage, 46
caruncle, 50
caseous, 60
cata-, 30
catalepsy, 18, 30
catalysis, 30, 85
cataract, 19
catarrh, 79
catatonia, 76
cauda, 46
causalgia, 75
causis, 75
caustices, 75
cautery, 21, 75
caverna, 52
cavities, 52–4
cavus, 65
cele, 19
cella, 46, 52
cent-, 62
centrifugal, 74
centripetal, 74
cephale, 46
cephalic, 96
cercos, 46
cerebellum, 51
cerebrospinal, 26
cerebrum, 46
cervix, 47
cestode, 74
cestos, 52
chaite, 69
chalasis, 77
chancre, 90, 104, 105
change, 78
Chaucer, Geoffrey, 3
cheilos, 46

cheir, 46
chemotherapy, 31
chezo, 84
chiasma, 48
chicle, 93
chiclero ulcer, 93
Chinese, 118
chiropodists, 110
chloros, 66
chlorosis, 111
choana, 48
cholagogue, 77
chole, 9, 11, 57
chole, melaina, 12
cholecystitis, 57
cholera, 39, 57, 79
cholesterol, 8, 9, 67
chondrion, 51
chondros, 46
chorea, 79
chorion, 54
choroid, 49
chroma, 65
chromaffin, 65
chromatophobe, 65
chromatophore, 78
chromosome, 11, 65
chronos, 75
chutta, 97
chylos, 57
chymos, 57
cicatrix, 69
cilia, 69
cingulum, 74
circadian, 75
circulation, 7
cirrhosis, 66
cirsoid, 49
cisterna, 52
clast-, 88
clastos, 85
claudication, 79
claustrophobia, 13
clavicula, 46
cleis, 46
climacteric, 17
clinic/clinical, 31
clinoid, 49
cloaca, 14
clonos, 79
clostridium, 52
cneme, 46

coarctation, 77
coccidium, 52
coccos (cuckoo), 58
coccos (berry), 59, 73
coccus, 52
coccyx, 48
cochlea, 48
coilia, 52
coitus, 74
colicos, 80
collagen, 60
colloid, 14, 49, 60
coloboma, 86
colon, 112–13
colour, 65–7
colpos, 46
coma, 82
comedo, 68
communications, 54–5
condyle, 19
condyloma, 19
conjugare, 74
Conn's syndrome, 100
construction, 84–5
contra, 70
contraction, 77
contre-coup, 90
Coomb's test, 100
copros, 58
cor, 47
coracoid, 49
corax, 58
cordial, 112
Coriolanus, 108
cornea, 15
corneus, 68
coronary, 59
corone, 58
coronoid, 49
corpus, 47
corpuscle, 51
cortex, 7
coryza, 12, 75
coxa, 46
Coxiella burnettii, 102
craniopagus, 74
craniotabes, 87
creas, 46
cremaster, 74
crepitare, 86
crepitation, 86

cretin, 21
cribriform, 50
cribrum, 14, 46
cricoid, 49
crinein, 74
crotos, 76
crus, 46
cryptorchidism, 75
cryptos, 75
cubitum, 46
cuboid, 49
cuirasse, en, 89–90
culebrilla, 98
cuneiform, 50
curette, 90
cuspis, 71
cutis, 46
cyanos, 66
cyanosis, 111
cyclitis, 64
cyesis, 83
cystis, 52
cystocele, 19

DACRYOCYSTITIS, 58
dacryon, 58
dactylos, 46
dandy, 93
Darmbrand, 95
death, 86
débridement, 90
dec-, 62
decay, 86
decem-, 62
decidua, 15, 80
deciduus, 80
decubitus, 72
decussate, 79
deficiency, 61
delphys, 46
deltoid, 49
demos, 70
De Motu Cordis, 4
dendrite, 73
dendron, 73
dengue, 93, 100
dens, 46
dentigerous, 26
derma, 46
dermatology, 26
desis, 74

desmoid, 49
desmos, 74
destruction, 85
detritus, 85
deuter-, 62
dhoti, 97
di-, 62
dia-, 30, 74
diadocho-, 76
diagnosis, 32
dialects, 114
diapedsis, 79
diaphoresis, 79
diaphragm, 13
diaphysis, 83
diarrhoea, 79
diastole, 72, 77
diathesis, 36, 72
dice, 20
dicrotic, 76
dictionaries, 103–4
didymi, 62
dies, 75
difficulty, 78
digestion, 83–4
digitus, 46
diminutives, 50
diphtheria, 55, 99
diphthongs, 116
diplo-, 63
diploe, 63
dipsa, 84
diseases, naming of, 32–5
distribution, 73–4
divertere, 78
diverticulosis, 35
diverticulum, 51, 78
DNA, 99
dochos, 52
doctor, 31
dolichocephalic, 64
doloureux, 92
dornase, 100
dose, 31
douche, 90
douloureux, 92
dromas, 79
ductus, 14, 54
Dunbar, William, 3
duodenum, 15, 112
dura mater, 67

dynamis, 76
dys-, 78
dyschezia, 84
dyscrasia, 81
dysentery, 78
dysgerminoma, 82
dysdiadochokinesis, 76
dyslalia, 82
dysmenorrhoea, 78, 79
dyspareunia, 83
dyspepsia, 78
dyspeptic, 84
dysphagia, 78, 84
dyspnoea, 56
dystrophy, 83

EASE, 78
eburnus, 67
ecchymosis, 57
echinos, 68
echo-virus, 100
eclampsia, 17
ecology, 71
ectasis, 77
ectopic, 72
ectropion, 78
eczema, 12, 75
editors, 38
efferent, 27
electron, 60
elephas, 59
elision, 26
elixir, 96
embolus, 27, 85
emeticos, 84
emollient, 67
empathy, 106
Empedocles, 20
emphysema, 77
empiric, 40
empyema, 57
encephalon, 46
encephalopathy, 105
en cuirasse, 89–90
endocrine, 74
endothelium, 18
enfermedad, 93
ennea-, 62
ensiform, 14, 50
enteron, 46
entoma, 58
entropion, 78

enuresis, 84
enzyme, 60
eos, 66
eosinophil, 66
ephebos, 70
epidemic, 70
epididymis, 43
epilepsy, 18, 30, 85
epiphora, 79
epiphysis, 83
epiploon, 46
epision, 46
espispadias, 55
epistaxis, 79
epithelium, 18
eponyms, 33, 100–2
Epstein-Barr virus, 100
epulis, 26
equus, 59
Erasistratus, 19
erepsin, 84
ergot, 90
erisipela de la Costa, 93
erotic, 22
erythema, 65
erythroblast, 82
erythros, 65
espundia, 93
essential, 34
ester, 95
ethmoid, 46, 49
eu-, 62
eugenic, 78
euphoria, 79
eurys, 64, 77
euthanasia, 78, 87
euthyroid, 78
exacerbate, 86
exanthem, 83
excess, 61–2
excoriare, 81
excretion, 83–4
expansion, 77
extensor, 76

F., 87
fabrics, 55–6
faex, 58
falciform, 50
falx, 14
farina, 60

fascia, 55, 73
fasciculus, 55
fauces, 13
favism, 92
favus, 68, 92
febris, 75
feeling, 80
fenestra, 54
fetus, 116
fever, 17
fibra, 55
fibrinogen, 36
fibroid, 49
fibula, 14
fievre boutonneuse, 90
filaria, 55
filariasis, 35
filum, 55
fimbria, 55
fistula, 14, 54
Fleckmilz, 95
flagellum, 51
flavus, 66
flocculus, 51, 55
fluids, 56–8
focus, 13
folie, 90
follicle, 51
folliculus, 52
fomites, 21
fontanelle, 14, 51
foramen, 54
form, 64–5
formalin, 81
forme fruste, 90
formica, 81
fornix, 14
fossa, 14
fovea, 53
fovimentum, 75
Fracastoro, Girolamo, 23
fracture, 6
fremitus, 86
French, 89–92
French disease, 105
French mole, 107
frenulum, 51
ft., 87
fugax, 76
fugere, 74
fundament, 113

INDEX

fungiform, 50
furunculus, 68
fusiform, 50

GALA, 57
galactose, 57
Galen, 11, 14, 106
galenical, 102
gamete, 70
gamma-camera, 110
gamma-globulin, 36
gammopathy, 36
gamos, 70
ganglion, 55
gangrene, 87
garg., 87
gargarizein, 86
gargle, 86
garrotter, 16
gaster, 53
gastric, 112
gemini, 63
genders, 42
gene-, 84
genetics, 70
genos, 70, 83
geriatrics, 71
German, 5, 94–5
germ-cell, 82
germen, 82
geron, 71
gestalt, 94
gestare, 83
gestation, 83
geusis, 81
Gitterzell, 95
glans, 45
glans penis, 46
glaucoma, 17, 66
glaucos, 66
glenoid, 16, 49
glia, 60
globin, 64
globus, 64
glomus, 55
glossa, 46
glotta, 46
glucose, 81
glus, glut-, 60
glycosuria, 81
glycys, 81
gnathos, 46

gnosia, 82
goitre, 90
gonad, 83
gonorrhoea, 83
goodness, 78
gout, 4, 34, 39
graft, 15
grand mal, 90
graphe, 82
Grave's disease, 101
gravidus, 83
gravity, 7
Greek/Latin
  synonyms, 45–7
Greek letters, x
Greek plurals, 41
Greek words in Latin, 24
grippe, 92
ground-nut poisoning, 99
growth, 82–3
gubernaculum, 48
guillotine, 90
gustatory, 81
gustus, 81
gut, 111–13
guttae, 87
guttar, 90
gynaecology, 71
gyne, 71
gyrus, 64

HABENULA, 51
hac nocte, 87
haem, 9
haemangioma, 51
haematemesis, 84
haematocele, 19
haematoporphyrin, 66
haemolysis,
haemoptysis, 84
haemorrhage, 79
haemorrhoids, 79
haemosiderosis, 35
haemostasis, 72
Hahnemann, Samuel, 106, 107
haima, 11, 46, 57
halitosis, 17, 56
halitus, 56
halzoun, 96

hamulus, 51
hamus, 48
haploid, 63
haptein, 74
hardness, 67
Harvey, William, 4, 5, 7, 11
haust., 87
haustrations, 48
haustrum, 48
HE, 99
hebe, 71, 88
hebephrenia, 71
hebes, 88
hect-, 62
helicotrema, 55
helix, 65
helminth, 48
hemera, 20
hemeralopia, 20
hemi-, 62
hemianopia, 81
hemicrania, 91
hemiplegia, 18
Henry V, King, 3
Henryson, Robert, 3
hept-, 62
hermaphrodite, 22
hernia, 21
herpes, 17, 79
heteros, 70
heterozygous, 63
hex-, 62
hiatus, 54
hidradenoma, 57
hidros, 57, 88
hilum, 48
"hippo", 107
hippocampus, 48, 59
Hippocrates, 10
hippus, 19
hirsutus, 68
histiocyte, 52
histion, 52
histology, 15, 55
histos, 52, 55
Hodgkin's disease, 101
homeopathy, 105–6
homo-, 69, 88
homoeo-, 69, 88
homozygous, 63
hormone, 77

humerus, 47
humoral theory, 11–12
hyalon, 74
hybrid words, 41–2
hydatid, 21
hydatiform, 107
hydor, 58, 88
hydro-, 88
hydrocele, 19, 116
hydropathy, 106
hygiene, 22, 32
hymen, 18, 23, 54
hyoid, 49
hyper-, 61, 107
hyperbaric, 67
hypercholesterol-
  aemia, 8
hypergammaglobulin-
  aemia, 36
hyperkryptonaemia, 9
hyperpiesis, 76
hyperplasia, 84
hyperpnoea, 11
hypertension, 32–3
hypertonic, 76
hypertrophy, 83
hyperuricaemia, 34
hypnos, 82
hypnotic, 82
hypo-, 61, 107
hypochondria, 12
hypocrite, 107
hypoglycaemia, 39
hypophysis, 82
hypopyon, 17–18
hypospadias, 55
hypothesis, 72
hystera, 46
hysteria, 12

-IA, 34
-iasis, 35
iatrogenic, 31, 84
iatros, 31
ichthyosis, 68
ichthys, 68
icterus, 66
identity, 69–70
idio-, 16
-*idion*, 52
idiopathic, 34, 69
idios, 69

idiosyncrasy, 69, 81
idiotes, 16
-idium, 52
-iform, 14, 50
ikteros, 111
ileum, 38, 65, 88, 112
ileus, 65, 112
ilium, 88
immunity, 86
impetere, 18
impetigo, 18, 85
incus, 14, 48
infarct, 85
influenza, 92
infundibulum, 48
inoculation, 15
intestines, 113
intestinus, 46
intravascular, 7, 8
involucrum, 53
ipse, 70
ipsilateral, 70
iris, 65
iron-mould, 107
irruption, 27
ischaemia, 86
ischion, 46
-ism, 34
-ismus, 34
iso-, 53
itai-itai-byo, 97
Italian, 92–3
itch, 109
iter, 54
-itis, 34

JAUNDICE, 32, 66,
  111
jaunisse, 111
jejunum, 15, 112
Jenner's vaccine, 106
jigger, 97
John, King, 3
John of Trevisa, 16
Johnson, Dr Samuel,
  104, 115
Jonson, Ben, 6
jugular, 63
juxta-aortic, 40

KALA-AZAR, 97
kalium, 60, 95

kangri, 97
karyokinesis, 59
karyon, 59
karyorrhexis, 79
keloid, 21
keratin, 61
keratitis, 68
keratos, 68
kernicterus, 95
kestus, 74
kilo-, 62
kinaesthesia, 78
kinema, 78
Koch's postulates, 100
koilonychia, 65
krauros, 67
kreatoelia, 107
kryos, 75
kuru, 97
kwashiorkor, 97–8
kyma, 80
kyphosis, 64

LABIUM, 46
lac, 57
lachrymal (gland), 57
lacrima, 57
lacteals, 57
lacuna, 53
Laennec, Réné, 91
lagophthalmos, 59
lagos, 59
lalis, 82
lambdoid, 49
lamella, 65
lamina, 65
Lancet, vii 115,
  116
Lao lao, 98
lapsus, 80
Lassa fever, 98
Latin, 3, 4, 5–6 *et
  passim*
Latin/Greek synonyms,
  45–7
Latin, Greek words in,
  24
latus, 64
lavage, 90
lecithos, 61
legionnaire's disease,
  91

leios, 68
Leishmania donovanii, 102
Leishmaniasis, 93, 94, 97
lemniscus, 55
lens, 48, 60
lentiform, 60
leo, 59
leontiasis, 59
lepra, 68
leprosy, 18, 68, 98
lepsis, 18, 85
leptos, 67
lesbianism, 23
lethargos, 82
leucopenia, 116
leucoplakia, 65
leucorrhoea, 79
leucos, 66
leukaemia, 100
leukocyte, 117
lexis, 82
libido, 80
lichen, 59
lien, 47
ligament, 74
ligare, 74
ligature, 74
limbus, 55
lingua, 46
lingula, 51
lipidosis, 35
lipoid, 49
lipos, 61
liq., 87
listhesis, 80
lithos, 61
lithotrite, 85
lobule, 51
locomotor, 72
locus, 72
loiasis, 98
longanon, 113
longus, 64
loqui, 86
lordosis, 64
lot., 87
lucidus, 75
lues, 85
lumbricus, 59
lumen, 15

luna, 64, 75
lunatic, 75
lupus, 21, 59
luteus, 66
Luther's Bible, 5
lympha, 57
lymphocytes, 57
lys-, 26
lysis, 85

MACERATE, 84
macros, 63
macula, 72
maculopapular, 39
Madura foot, 98
maduromycosis, 98
Magenstrasse, 95
magnus, 63
main en griffe, 91
major, 63
malabsorption, 78
malacos, 67
malaria, 92
malleolus, 51
malleus, 14, 48
malus, 78
mamma, 46
mammilliform, 50
mandere, 84
mandible, 84
mandibulum, 46
mane, 87
manometer, 67
manubrium, 48
manus, 46
marasmus, 87
masochism, 102
massage, 91
masseter, 84
mast cell, 95
mastoid, 49
mastopathy, 105
mastos, 46
mater, 96
maxilla, 46
maximus, 63
meaning, changes of, 40
measurements, 63
meatus, 54
meconium, 60
mediastinum, 54

medicine, 4, 31
medicine, ancient, 10–13
medulla, 46, 73
megakaryocyte, 59
megalos, 63
megrim, 91
melaena, 15
melaina chole, 12
melancholic, 12
melanoma, 66
melas, 66
membrana, 54
membranes, 54
mene, 75
meninges, 54
meningitis, 35
meningocele, 19
menis, 75
meniscus, 64
menopause, 75
menorrhagia, 80
mens, ment-, 81, 88
menses, 75, 88
menstrual, 75
mental states, 81–2
mercury, 66
merycism, 84
mesothelium, 18
meta-, 30, 31, 78
metabolism, 85
metamorphosis, 78
metaplasia, 78
metastasis, 78
meteorism, 77
methaemoglobin, 26, 78
metra, 46
metron, 63
metrorrhagia, 80
micros, 63
migraine, 91
miliary tuberculosis, 60
milli-, 62
milium, 60
Milton, John, 6
minimus, 63
minor, 63
miscegenation, 70
mist., 87
mitochrondria, 51

mitos, 56
mitosis, 56
mitte, 87
Mkar disease, 98
mnemonic, 82
mnesis, 82
modification, 78
molar, 84
mole, 107, 108
mollis, 67
molluscus, 67
mongolism, 98
moniliasis, 65
mono-, 62
monoplegia, 18
morbid, 40
morbilli, 17
moros, 82
morphe, 23, 64
morphia, 23, 64
morula, 51
mosquito, 93
mouldiwarp, 107
movement, 78–80
Much Ado, 108–9
mucin, 57
mucus, 57, 88
'mule rule', 33
munitis, 86
Murray, Sir James, 115
musca, 59, 93
musculus, 46
myces, 60, 88
mycology, 60
mydriatic, 21
myelin, 73
myeloma, 73
myelos, 46
mylos, 84
myopia, 17
myotatic, 77
mys-, myo-, 46, 59
myxa, 57, 88
myxoedema, 57
myxoma, 57

NAEVUS, 69, 107–8
naphtha, 95
narce, 82
narcissism, 23
narcotic, 82
nasus, 47
natrium, 61, 95
Natural Spirit, 11
nausea, 18
navicula, 51
necrosis, 87
nectere, 74
nema, 56
nematode, 56
neonatorum, 83
neoplastic, 104
neos, 82
nephropathy, 105
nephropexy, 74
nephros, 46
nephrosis, 5
nervus, 46
neuralgia, 60, 80
neurilemma, 26, 73
neuroblastoma, 82
neurology, 13
neuron, 13, 46
New Eng. J. Med., 115
New Guinea pidgin, 114
Newton, Sir Isaac, 7
nictare, 80
niger, 66
nocere, 86
noct-, 25
nocte, 87
nocturia, 25
nodule, 51
noiein, 82
non-anglophones, 39
Norman-French, 3, 6
novem-, 62
nox, noct-, 75
nucha, 96
nucleolus, 51, 60
nucleus, 51, 60
numbers, 62
nummus, 65
nutrition, 83–4
nux, nuc-,
nyctalopia, 20, 75
nymphe, 71
nystagmus, 19, 80
nyx, nyct-, 20, 75

OBSTETRICS, 72
obstruction, 85
obturator, 85
occiput, 27
occultus, 75
oct-, 62
odont-, 25
odontoid, 2, 49
odous, odont-, 46
odyne, 80
O.E.D, viii, 104, 113
oedema, 77
oedipal, 117
Oedipus complex, 23
oesophagus, 111, 117
oestrus, 17
-oid, 9, 14, 49
oidema, 77
oidium, 52
oikos, 71
-ol, 9
Old English, 3
olere, 81
olfactory, 81
oligos, 61
Oliver Twist, 106
-oma, 35
omentum, 46
omos, 47
omphalos, 46
onchocerciasis, 93
oncology, 82
oncornavirus, 100
oncos, 83
On the Circulation of the Blood, 5
ontogenesis, 71
Onyalai, 98
O-nyong-nyong, 98, 100
onyx, 47
oon, 47, 52
openings, 54–5
operculum, 54
ophthalmos, 47
opisthen, 64
opsonin, 84
optic, 81
oral, 54
orbis, 64
orchidectomy, 26
orchis, 47
orexis, 84
organon, 47

ortho-, 30
orthopaedics, 8, 32, 64, 109
orthopnoea, 56, 64
orthopod, 109–10
orthopodos, 110
orthos, 64, 109
os, or-, 47, 54, 88
os, oss-, 47, 88
os innominatum, 21
-osis, 35
osme, 81
osmos, 79
ossicle, 51
osteo-, 88
osteoblast, 82
osteoclastic, 85
osteolytic, 85
osteomalacia, 67
osteon, 47
osteopathy, 106
ostium, 54, 88
ouron, 58
ous, otos, 47
ovarium, 47
ovum, 47
oxyntic, 81
oxys, 65, 76, 81
oxytocin, 83
oxyuris, 65

PABULUM, 84
pachys, 67
paederasty, 71
paediatrics, 32, 71
paedomorphic, 117
pagos, 74
pais, paid-, 71, 88, 109
pallidus, 66
palpebra, 46
pampiniform, 50
pan-, 61
panacea, 23
panniculus, 56
pannus, 56
para-, 14, 30, 31, 78
Paracelsian, 102
paraesthesia, 80
paratyphoid, 14
parameter, 30, 118
paranoia, 82
paraplegia, 18, 85

parasite, 83
parathormone, 27
Paré, Ambroise, 19
paregoreo, 80
parenchyma, 19
parere, 83
paresis, 77
pareunos, 83
paries, pariet-, 54
parietal, 54
parkinsonian, 101
paroxysm, 76
parthenos, 71
partitions, 54
parvus, 63
PAS, 99
pasteurization, 101
patella, 53
pathogenic, 84
pathognomonic, 32
pathological, 40
pathologikos, 106
pathos, 106
-pathy, 35, 105–6
patulus, 54
p.c., 87
pecten, 48
pectoriloquy, 86
pectus, 86
ped-, 25
pedesis, 79
pedicle, 51
pediculus, 51, 58
peduncle, 51
pella, 46
pellagra, 85, 93
pemphigus, 68
pemphis, 68
pen, 61
penicillia, 14
penis, 47
pent-, 62
pepsis, 84
Pepys, Samuel, 6
peristalsis, 21
peri-thymic, 40
peritoneum, 76
peritonitis, 32
perone, 47
peroneus, 14
pertussis, 39, 86

pes, ped-, 47, 88
pessary, 64
pessos, 64
petechia, 93
petere, 74
petit mal, 90
petri dish, 101
petrous, 67
pexis, 74
phaeos, 66
phagedaena, 69
phagein, 84
phakos, 60
phalanx, 14
phallos, 47
pharmacy, 31
phasis, 82
phimosis, 77
phlebography, 41
phlegm, 11
phlegma, 11
phlegmatic, 19
phleps, phleb, 47
phlyctaina, 68
phobos, 81
Phoenix, 17
phone, 82
phonetic spelling, 117
phora, 78
phoreo, 79
phos, phot-, 81
photopathy, 106
photophobia, 81
photo-sensitive, 81
phragma, 54
phren, 81
phrenic, 12
phryne, 59, 68
phrynoderma, 68
phthiriasis, 35
phthisis, 87
phylaxis, 86
phylogenesis, 71
phylon, 71
phyma, 69
physic, 31
physical, 31
physician, 4, 31
physicist, 31
physiology, 31
physiotherapy, 31
physis, 82

phyton, 59
pibloktu, 98
picornavirus, 100
pidgin, 114
piedra, 93
piesis, 76
pigbel, 98
pilus, 69
pineal, 48
pinna, 48
pinta, 94
pisiform, 50
pituitary, 12
pityron, 68
placebo, 80
plague, 18
plants, 59–60
plasma, 57, 84
plast-, 98
plastic, 85
Plato, 19–20
platysma, 65
plax, 65
plege, 18, 85
pleion, 62
plethora, 61
pleurisy, 4, 34
pleurodynia, 80
plexus, 56
plica, 56
Plummer-Vinson's disease, 101
plurals, 41, 42, 43–4
pneuma, 10, 11, 56
pneumoconiosis, 60
pneumogastric, 56
pneumon, 47
pneumonia, 11, 34, 56
pneumonitis, 35
pnoe, 56
podagra, 34, 85
poiesis, 85
poikilo-, 63
poison, 4
poliomyelitis, 66, 73
polios, 66
poly-, 62
polycythaemia, 26, 118
polydipsia, 84
pompholyx, 68
poros, 54
porphyra, 66

position, 71–2
pous, pod-, 47, 109
praecox, 76
prandium, 84
praxis, 82
precocity, 76
prefixes, 27–9
presbys, 71
priapism, 23
prim-, 62
primaquine sensitivity, 92
primary, 34
primipara, 83
p.r.n., 87
procidentia, 80
proctos, 47
prognosis, 32
prolapse, 80
prophylaxis, 86
proprioceptive, 69
proprius, 69
prostate, 72
prosthesis, 72
prot-, 62
prurigo, 81
prurire, 81
psammos, 61
pseudo-, 14, 50
pseudocyesis, 50
pseudoleukaemia, 50
pseudomembranous, 50
psittacos, 59
psora, 81
psyche, 10, 11, 81
psychiatry, 11
psychology, 11, 23
psychros, 75
pterygoid, 49
ptoma, 87
ptosis, 80
ptyalin, 84
ptysis, 84
pubis, 46, 71
pudenda, 17
puer, 71
puerperium, 71
pulex, 58
pulmo, 47
pulvinar, 56
P.U.O., 17

pupil, 16
purpurus, 66
pyaemia, 57
pycnos, 73
pyelos, 47, 53
pyknosis, 73
pylorus, 13, 95
pyo-, 57
pyon, 57
pyr, 75, 88
pyr-, 88
pyreticos, 75
pyrexia, 17, 75
pyriform, 50

Q.S., 87
quadr-, 62
quadrigemina, 63
quantity, 61–2
quarantine, 93
Quiller-Couch, Sir Arthur, 41
quinine, 94
quinqu-, 62
quinsy, 16
quotidian, 75

R, 23
rabies, 85
racemos, 73
rad, 100
radar, 110
râle, 91
ramus, 73
rana, 59
ranula, 59
raster, 111
receptacles, 52–4
rectum, 64, 113
rectus, 64
regimen, 100
relations, 70–1
relaxation, 76–7
rem, 100
ren, 46
Renaissance, 5
reovirus, 100
rep, 100
rep., 87
rep, ambo., 87
rep. omnia, 88
reproduction, 82–3

INDEX

resemblance, 48–50
restiform, 50
rete, 56
retention, 6
reticulum, 56
retrovirus, 100
rhabdos, 65
rhachis, 47
rhachitis, 21
rhagades, 69
rhagia, 79
rhaphe, 74
rhesus, 59
rheum, 12
rheuma, 79
rheumatic fever, 12
rheumatism, 12, 36, 79
rheumatoid arthritis, 12
rhexis, 26, 79
rhinophyma, 69
rhis, rhin-, 47
rhodopsin, 66
rhoia, 79
rhonchos, 86
rhonchus, 86
rhythmos, 76
Richard II, King, 3
rickets, 21, 88
rickettsia, 88
Rickettsia prowazeki, 102
rigor, 76
rima, 54
RNA, 99
roseus, 66
rotundus, 64
rubella, 65
rubeola, 65
ruber, 65
rubro-spinal tract, 66
ruga, 56, 68

SACCULE, 51
sacculus, 53
sacrum, 15
sadism, 102
St Anthony's Fire, 23
St Vitus's Dance, 23
salpinx, 14
sanguine, 12, 57
sanguis, 46, 57

saphenes, 75
saprophyte, 59
sapros, 87
sartorius, 15
sarx, sarc-, 46
Saxons, 114
scabere, 81, 109
scabies, 39, 81, 108–9
scabs, 108–9
scalenos, 65
scan, 110–11
scandere, 110
scaphoid, 49
schistosomiasis, 35
schizein, 74
schizophrenia, 74
science, 31
scirrhous, 67
sclera, 67
sclerosis, 67
scoliosis, 64
scopos, 81
scotomos, 66
scrub typhus, 99
scybalon, 58
sebum, 61
sec. art., 88
secund-, 62
sella, 48
semen, 83
semi-, 62
senex, 71
senna, 96
sensation, 80, 81
senses, special, 81
separation, 74
sepsis, 87
sept-, 62
septum, 13, 54
sequestrum, 87
serpiginous, 79
serum, 57
sesamoid, 49
sex-, 62
Shakespeare, William, 3, 6, 108, 109
shape, 64–5
shingles, 74
sialon, 57
siccus, 68
sideros, 61
sigmoid, 49, 113

silicosis, 35
sinus, 53, 54
Sir Gawain and the Green Knight, 3
sitos, 83
situs, 72
size, 63
skabb, 109
skeletos, 68
smegma, 61
softness, 67
soma, 10, 11, 47
somatic, 11
somnos, 82
sopor, 82
s.o.s., 88, 99
soufflé, 91
spadion, 55
Spanish, 93–4
spasm, 76
spastic, 77
speed, 76
speira, 65
spermatozoa, 83
sphenoid, 49
sphincter, 14
sphygmomanometer, 76
sphyxis, 76
spina, 47
Spirit, Animal, Natural, Vital, 11
spirochaete, 69
spissus, 67
splanchna, 47
spleen, 12
splen, 47
spondylos, 47
spongioblast, 56
spongos, 56
sporadic, 83
spore, 83
sporos, 83
squama, 68
ss, 88
stapes, 14, 48
staphylococcus, 59
staphylos, 73
stasis, 72
stat-, 26
statistics, 72
staxis, 79

stearic, 61
steatorrhoea, 61
stella, 65
stems, 25–6
stenosis, 64, 77
-ster-, 9
stercus, 58
stereognosis, 67
stereos, 67
steroids, 9
stertere, 86
stertorous, 86
stethos, 47
sthenos, 77
stigma, 72
stimulation, 77
stole, 72
stoma, 47, 55, 112
stomach, 112
streptococcus, 73
streptos, 73
stria, 53
stroma, 53
strongylos, 64
styloid, 14, 49
styptic, 77
substances, 60–1
sudor, 57
suffixes, 29
sugar, 95
sulcus, 53
suppurate, 57
surface, 68
surgeon, 4
surgery, 31
sustentaculum, 48
sycosis, 60
sympathetic, 13
sympathy, 106
symphysis, 74
symposium, 19
symptom, 30, 80
syn-, 74
synapse, 74
syncope, 86
syncrasis, 81
syncytium, 73
syndrome, 30, 79
synechiae, 74
synonyms, 45–7
synostosis, 74
synovia, 61

synthesis, 85
syphilis, 23, 96
Syphilis, 24
syr., 88
syrinx, 48
syrup, 96
systole, 27, 72, 74, 77

TAB., 88
tabes, 87
tache, 91
tachycardia, 76
tachys, 76
tactus, 81
taenia, 48, 56
tainia, 56
talipes, 80
talus, 20
tampion, 91
tampon, 91
tanapox, 98
tapes, 56
tapetum, 56
tarsus, 19
tasis, 77
taxis, 72
t.d.s., 88
tectorium, 48
tegmentum, 53
teino, 76
teirein, 85
telangiectasis, 72
telepathy, 106
telos, 72
temperature, 75
temple, 21
temporal, 21
tendo, 47
tendo Achillis, 24
tendon, 76
tenesmus, 76
tenon, 47
tension, 76–7
tensor, 76
tentorium, 48
ter-, 62
teras, 83
teratoma, 83
teres, 64
tert-, 62
testis, 47
tetanus, 76

tetany, 76
tetr-, 62
texture, 55–6
thalassaemia, 8
thanatos, 87
theca, 53
thele, 18
theloma, 107
thenar, 15
therapy, 31
-therapy, 106
therme, 75
thesis, 72
thetos, 72
thickness, 67
thinness, 67
thorax, 17, 47
thrombos, 85
thymos, 21–2, 80
thymus, 21–2
thyroid, 49
tibia, 48
tic, 91
tic douloureux, 91–2
tick-bite fever, 90
t.i.d., 88, 99
time, 75–6
tinct., 88
tinnere, 86
tinnitus, 86
tissue, 91
tocos, 83
tome, 26
topography, 72
topos, 72
torcula, 14
tormina, 80
torticollis, 65
trancazo, 92
transliteration, x
transport, 36
trapezoid, 50
trauma, 86
trechein, 79
trema, 55

trabeculum, 13, 43
trachea, 68
trachelos, 47
trachoma, 68

trepanon, 65
treponema, 65
tresis, 55
tri-, 62
triceps, 46
trichos, 69
tricuspid, 71
trigeminal, 63
trigone, 65
triquetrum, 65
trismus, 84
trit-, 62
trocar, 91
troch., 88
trochanter, 79
trochlea, 48, 79
trochos, 79
trop-, 88
troph-, 88
trophe, 83
tropos, 26, 78
trypanosome, 65
trypanosomiasis, 35
TSH, 99
tsutsugamushi, 99
tubercle, 51
tuberculosis, 35
tumours, 35
tunica, 53
turbinate, 65
tussis, 86
Twelfth Night, 108
Tyler, Wat, 3
typanites, 86
tympanum, 14, 49, 86
tyndalization, 101
typhoid, 14, 50
typhus, 14, 17

UMBILICUS, 46, 49, 51, 104
un-, 62
unciform, 50
unguis, 47
urea, 58
ureter, 58
urethra, 58
urine, 58
uta, 94
uterus, 46
utricle, 51
urticaria, 60
urea, 60
uvula, 51, 60, 73

VACCINATION, 15
vagina, 46, 53
vagus, 79
valgus, 20, 74
variable, 40
varicella, 68
varicocele, 77
variola, 68
varioliform, 39
varius, 68
varix, 77
varus, 74
vas, 53
vascular, 51
veld(t) sore, 99
vena, 47
venereal, 24
venography, 41
venter, 53, 112
ventral, 112
ventricle, 51
vermiform, 14
vernacular, 2, 39
vertebra, 47
verruca, 69
verruga peruana, 94
veru, 71
verumontanum, 71
vesicular, 51
vestibulum, 54
via, 14

villus, 69
violence, 85–6
virus, 86
viscera, 47
viscus, 47
visibility, 74–5
Vital Spirit, 11
vitellus, 61
vitreous humour, 75
vitrum, 75
vomer, 14, 49
vowels, linking, 26
vulva, 54

WASTING, 86
Webster, Noah, 104, 115, 117
Websterisms, 115–16
weight, 67
whooping cough, 39
word-formation, rules of, 41–4
Wyclif's Bible, 4

XANTHOS, 66
xeroderma, 68
xeros, 68
xiphoid, 50
xylon, 61

YELLOW FEVER, 39, 100

ZEEIN, 12, 75
zoe, 56
zoon, 58
zoster, 74
zygoma, 63
zygon, 63
zygote, 63
zyme, 60
zymotic, 60